NOVA SCOTIA

A Health System Profile

Despite notable variation in health care policy from province to province, most scholarship published on the health care system in Canada uses a broad national perspective. Focusing on the health care systems of individual Canadian provinces and territories, this new Provincial and Territorial Health System Profiles series examines the social, political, economic, and epidemiological context of health care policy in each Canadian jurisdiction.

Turning a critical eye to the health care system in Nova Scotia, author Katherine Fierlbeck outlines the organizational and regulatory frameworks structuring provincial health care, while providing a detailed assessment of Nova Scotia's health financing, physical infrastructure, and service provision, and the efficacy of technological resources used in data tracking and health quality assessments. Structured for ease of comparison with other volumes in the series, *Nova Scotia: A Health System Profile* will help scholars draw analytic evidence-based policy conclusions about the health system of Nova Scotia and other Canadian provinces and territories.

(Provincial and Territorial Health System Profiles)

KATHERINE FIERLBECK is McCulloch Professor of Political Science at Dalhousie University.

Provincial and Territorial Health System Profiles

SERIES EDITOR: Gregory P. Marchildon, Director of the North American Observatory on Health Systems and Policies

This series of provincial and territorial health system profiles is sponsored and directed by the North American Observatory on Health Systems and Policies, a collaborative partnership of academic researchers, governments, and health organizations promoting evidence-informed health policy decision-making.

NOVA SCOTIA

A HEALTH SYSTEM PROFILE

Katherine Fierlbeck

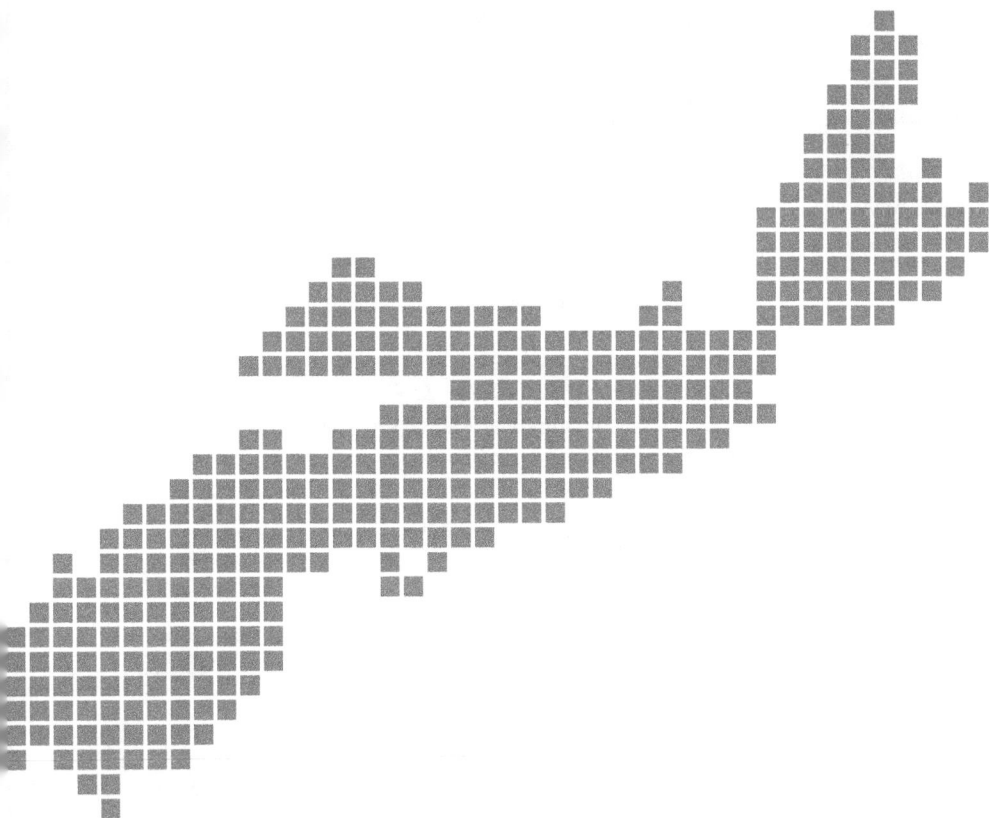

UNIVERSITY OF TORONTO PRESS
Toronto Buffalo London

© University of Toronto Press 2018
Toronto Buffalo London
utorontopress.com

ISBN 978-1-4875-0274-4 (cloth)   ISBN 978-1-4875-2214-8 (paper)

Library and Archives Canada Cataloguing in Publication

Fierlbeck, Katherine, author
Nova Scotia : a health system profile / Katherine Fierlbeck.

(Provincial and territorial health system profiles)
Includes bibliographical references and index.
ISBN 978-1-4875-0274-4 (cloth).   ISBN 978-1-4875-2214-8 (paper)

1. Medical care – Nova Scotia.   2. Medical policy – Nova Scotia.
I. Title.   II. Series: Provincial and territorial health system profiles

RA410.55.C35F54 2018   362.109716   C2018-900129-1

NORTH AMERICAN
OBSERVATORY
on Health Systems and Policies

This series of provincial and territorial health system profiles is sponsored and directed by the North American Observatory on Health Systems and Policies, a collaborative partnership of academic researchers, governments, and health organizations promoting evidence-informed health policy decision-making.

University of Toronto Press acknowledges the financial assistance to its publishing program of the Canada Council for the Arts and the Ontario Arts Council, an agency of the Government of Ontario.

Canada Council   Conseil des Arts
for the Arts   du Canada

ONTARIO ARTS COUNCIL
CONSEIL DES ARTS DE L'ONTARIO
an Ontario government agency
un organisme du gouvernement de l'Ontario

Funded by the   Financé par le
Government   gouvernement
of Canada   du Canada

Canadä

Contents

Figures, Tables, and Boxes

Figures

Boxes

Series Editor's Foreword

There is not, and has never been, a single Canadian health system. As subnational jurisdictions in one of the most decentralized federations in the world, provincial and territorial governments are the principle stewards for publicly financed health services and coverage in Canada. This makes it very difficult to describe the "Canadian system," much less compare Canada's system to national health systems in the rest of the world.

These were the key challenges I faced when I researched and wrote the two editions of the *Health Systems in Transition (HiT)* study on Canada for the European Observatory on Health Systems and Policies and the World Health Organization (Marchildon, 2006, 2013). The *HiT* template was prepared for the comparative review of national health systems (Rechl, Thomson, & van Ginnekan, 2010). In order to generalize at the pan-Canadian level of analysis, I was forced to make a number of adjustments and compromises.

This experience convinced me that a series of provincial and territorial health system profiles would be of great utility to decision makers, providers, scholars, and students alike. I experimented with adapting the *HiT* template to the provincial context with an initial profile of the Saskatchewan health system (Marchildon & O'Fee, 2007). This was followed a few years later by a profile of Nunavut based on a two-year study of the health system of that vast northern Canadian territory (Marchildon & Torgerson, 2013).

In 2013, I began looking for lead authors to take on the task of researching and writing individual provincial and territorial health system profiles. The University of Toronto Press agreed to publish the series on the understanding that the content would eventually be made freely available after the first year of publication through the North American Observatory on Health Systems and Policies (NAO). The purpose of the NAO is to examine and compare health systems and policies across jurisdictions, principally at the provincial and state level.

Each volume in this series focuses on the system and policies within an individual province or territory. A subject-matter template was developed requiring a diamond-hard focus on the jurisdiction in question – a single case study – with some compulsory data tables and figures putting that jurisdiction in a more pan-Canadian context. This case-study approach, relying heavily on the grey literature, is essential given the lack of any extensive secondary literature on the health systems and policies in most jurisdictions. The intent of this series is to provide a base line for future scholarly work and to encourage the development of a richer comparative literature on provincial and territorial health systems and policies.

Templates of the sort used in this series must also be flexible enough to allow authors the flexibility to focus on areas that may be unique to the jurisdiction in question. As a consequence, individual volume authors were encouraged to go beyond the template as long as they could keep the length of the profile reasonable. In addition, the provinces and territories vary considerably in size – both population and geography – and both fiscal and administrative capacity. These facts also speak to allowing some flexibility within the template. In the end, however, target lengths were set for the volumes with one principle in mind: to achieve a comfortable balance between studies that are concise enough to be of use to busy decision makers and providers but still detailed enough to be of utility for scholars and students.

Although provincial and territorial systems are nested within a pan-Canadian system in which the federal government as well as intergovernmental agencies can play an important role, authors were asked to focus on their particular provincial or territorial system. For example, the Canada Health Act and the federal hospital and medical care legislation that preceded it were instrumental in shaping provincial and territorial "Medicare" regulatory and policy approaches. However, there are important variations in provincial and territorial Medicare laws, policies, and approaches across Canada, and these have not been adequately described, much less compared. The profiles in this series will provide a foundation for future scholars to make analytic comparisons and draw evidence-based policy conclusions.

Those readers interested in a national health system study or federal policy initiatives and structures are encouraged to use the existing *HiT* study on Canada. This study is periodically updated and is freely available on the NAO website and should be treated as a contributing volume in the series.[1] This approach avoids repetition among individual volumes while economizing on the page length of each book.

It is important to note that the data tables required of all the provincial-territorial studies rely heavily on two very different sources. The first are the data held by the Canadian Institute for Health Information, an organization that has put considerable effort into ensuring that administrative and financial data have been defined and collected in ways that make it comparable. The second are the data from provincial and territorial ministries of health. Here, we can make few guarantees of comparability across jurisdictions, although the authors have been asked to be as precise as possible about the meaning assigned to terms by individual governments.

Each volume in this series has been put through the University of Toronto Press's peer-review process. While this has lengthened the time to publication – a significant factor in contemporary policy studies of this type – we felt that the importance of peer review outweighed the cost of the time involved. Moreover, we felt that these volumes contain much that is of permanent value, and therefore publishing through a highly reputable academic publisher would ensure longevity in a way that cannot be matched by relying solely on web-based, electronic dissemination. Indeed, in our unique arrangement with the University of Toronto Press, we hope we have achieved the best of two worlds: the high scholarly standards that come with traditional academic publication *and* the widest possible dissemination that comes with Internet-based distribution one year after paper publication.

It is my hope that these studies will form the essential foundation for future comparative health system and policy study in Canada. They should be seen as a place for researchers to begin their case study or comparative health systems and policy research. No doubt we will refine and improve the template for future editions of these provincial and territorial profiles, so we encourage your feedback.

Katherine Fierlbeck has produced this health system profile of Nova Scotia. I am indebted to her for putting aside almost two years of her time to research and write this volume. As the author of a citizen's guide to health care in Canada and a long-time student of health politics and policy, Professor Fierlbeck was the ideal individual to write this book.

---

1 http://ihpme.utoronto.ca/research/research-centres-initiatives/nao/.

Fortunately, this work turned out to be a fascinating process of discovery for her. She detected some unique details about Nova Scotia's health system, including the fact that the single-payer medical care coverage system in that province has been implemented and managed through a public-private organization that was an outgrowth of private insurance carriers. We can all learn much from her book.

Gregory P. Marchildon, Series Editor
Professor and Ontario Research Chair in Health Policy
and System Design
Institute of Health Policy, Management and Evaluation
University of Toronto

REFERENCES

Marchildon, G.P. (2006). *Health systems in transition: Canada.* Copenhagen: WHO Regional Office for Europe on behalf of the European Observatory on Health Systems and Policies. Subsequently published by the University of Toronto Press in 2007.

Marchildon, G.P. (2013). *Health systems in transition: Canada (2nd ed.).* Copenhagen: WHO Regional Office for Europe on behalf of the European Observatory on Health Systems and Policies. Simultaneously published by the University of Toronto Press in 2013.

Marchildon, G.P., & O'Fee, K. (2007). *Health care in Saskatchewan: An analytical profile.* Regina: Canadian Plains Research Center.

Marchildon, G.P., & Torgerson, R. (2013). *Nunavut: A health system profile.* Montreal: McGill-Queen's University Press.

Rechl, B., Thomson, S., & van Ginnekan, E. (2010). *Health systems in transition: Template for authors.* Copenhagen: WHO Regional Office for Europe on behalf of the European Observatory on Health Systems and Policies. Accessed on January 15, 2017: http://www.euro.who.int/__data/assets/pdf_file/0003/127497/E94479.pdf?ua=1

Preface and Acknowledgments

Studying health policy requires three levels of investigation. The first level is purely empirical: before we can make any assumptions, we must first gather whatever relevant data is available. As P.D. James was fond of reminding her readers, it never pays to theorize in advance of the facts. This point may seem rather obvious, but a disconcertingly large amount of health policy – such as the regionalization of centralized systems or the consolidation of decentralized ones – has been made based upon theoretical presuppositions of what ought to occur rather than what actually does.

The second level of investigation is causal and linear. Once we are able to ascertain what, in fact, is happening, the question that naturally comes next is *why*. Here policy studies have looked to the natural sciences, where the focus is on isolating the relationships between discrete variables. To understand how something works, we must convincingly be able to identify the causal pathways that link X and Y. To be convincing, the evidence of causality must be comprehendible, predictable, and replicable. Confidence in causal explanations underlies the "evidence-based medicine" approach, which itself is a key component of much rhetoric underlying health policy. Yet transcribing causal certainty to the policy domain is harder than it looks. The problem with putting human agents under the microscope is that it is devilishly difficult to determine pathways of causality in decision making. Health care, like other systems based on human interactions, becomes a sphere of causal complexity comprising multitudinous other spheres of causal complexity.

Recognizing this complexity, the third level of health policy analysis is iterative and contextual. Any changes in one part of a system may have unanticipated and possibly even profound consequences in others. These changes may even affect the initial agent of change in a recursive manner so that the causal relationship remains a highly dynamic one. In a linear analysis, "confounders" are to be isolated and eliminated; in a multilinear policy analysis, confounders themselves become relevant variables. The difficulty, of course, is in determining the precise force of any one variable over the others. This iterative relationship is also true of researchers' attempts to understand their world, for determination of what constitutes "valid" data can itself be a product of the way in which researchers have been trained to investigate their respective fields. The intellectual context within which researchers collect and interpret evidence is often as important as the raw data itself.

What this means is that health policy, as a discipline, cannot remain divided into the two solitudes defined by health services researchers, on the one hand, and social science researchers, on the other. The hard work of interpreting and understanding why things happen as they do within health systems is best undertaken using the well-honed tools of more than one discipline. This book is designed to be used by researchers across the disciplines, as well as by decision makers themselves. The purpose of the book is largely empirical: it merely aims to present information on how the system works and to provide a foundation for more analytical investigation. Yet even the simple collection of information in an intricate and ever-changing system is challenging. I have been incredibly fortunate to have had a considerable amount of feedback from academics, administrators, and practitioners who are profoundly knowledgeable about the health care system in Nova Scotia. I am deeply grateful for their advice. It is instructive to note that, much like the blind men describing the elephant, the "reality" of the system differs considerably depending on the particular part of the system with which each person is most intimately familiar. I have attempted to fuse this *Rashomon*-like presentation of information into a single narrative, but the result may be something that some of those I have consulted do not recognize (for example, where provincial figures were not identical to those of Canadian Institute for Health Information (CIHI) or Statistics Canada due to methodological differences, national figures were used so that they could be compared more easily to the statistics used in the companion volumes in this series). For this reason, the responsibility for the final product is mine and mine alone. Having made this disclaimer, there are many individuals whom I would like to thank for their time and for their feedback. These include Yukiko Asada, Vijay Bhasyakarla, Louise

Carbert, Keith Dares, Gordon Forsyth, Christine Gibbons, James Houston, Bill Lahey, Adrian Levy, Maureen MacDonald, Katie Mallam, Tom Marrie, Kevin McNamara, Jennifer Murdoch, Jock Murray, Jill Petrella, Hilda Power, Jeff Scott, Ingrid Sketris, Ron Stewart, and David Zitner. The Department of Health and Wellness was very gracious in responding to my numerous and detailed queries about how things worked. I would also like to thank the three anonymous reviewers for their constructive insights and comments. And, finally, I would like to thank Greg Marchildon, who somehow has the knack of being both intellectually critical and generously supportive at the very same time.

Acronyms

AART	Atlantic Assisted Reproductive Therapies
CCA	continuing care assistant
CDHA	Capital District Health Authority
CEC	collaborative emergency centre (also collaborative emergency care)
CHB	community health board
CHT	Canada Health Transfer
CIHI	Canadian Institute for Health Information
CIHR	Canadian Institutes of Health Research
COHP	Children's Oral Health Program
CPERS	Canadian Patient Experience Reporting System
DHA	district health authority
DHW	Department of Health and Wellness
DIS	Drug Information System
EHR	electronic health record
EHS	Emergency Health Services
EMC	Emergency Medical Care
EMR	electronic medical record
GDP	gross domestic product
HANS	Health Association of Nova Scotia
HHR	health human resources
HITS-NS	Health Information Technology Services Nova Scotia
HTA	health technology assessment
ICES	Institute for Clinical Evaluative Sciences (Ontario)
INAC	Indigenous and Northern Affairs Canada
IT	information technology

MHSA	Maritime Hospital Service Association
MMC	Maritime Medical Care
MOCINS	Model of Care Initiative in Nova Scotia
MSI	Medical Services Insurance
NSGEU	Nova Scotia Government and General Employees' Union
NSHA	Nova Scotia Health Authority
NShIS	Nova Scotia hospital Information System
NSNU	Nova Scotia Nurses' Union
NSPMP	Nova Scotia Prescription Monitoring Program
OECD	Organisation for Economic Cooperation and Development
OOP	out of pocket
P3	public-private partnership
PACS	Picture Archiving Communication System
PERS	Patient Experience Reporting System
PHAC	Public Health Agency of Canada
PHR	personal health record
RHA	regional health authority
RHB	regional health board
WHO	World Health Organization

NOVA SCOTIA

Chapter One

Introduction and Overview

That we can think of Canadian health care as a national "system" is largely due to the fact that Canada's provinces are very similar in the way that they tend to finance, provide, and regulate health care services (Marchildon, 2013; Fierlbeck, 2011 & 2016). Yet each province possesses considerable autonomy in determining the particular shape of its respective health care system. There is a national presence in health care through legislative jurisdiction (the federal government, for example, is responsible for the regulation of pharmaceuticals, assisted dying, and assisted human reproduction) and through the conditions attached to the transfer of health care funding. Federal financial support to provinces for health care is in practice more a political convention than a direct constitutional obligation. The principal framework for federal financial support has been the Canada Health Act 1984 (which consolidated two previous federal legislative acts, the 1957 Hospital Insurance and Diagnostic Services Act and the 1966 Medical Care Act), although there are also some bilateral financial health agreements between Ottawa and the provinces. The proportion of provincial health spending that comes from the federal government varies through time and across provinces, but generally averages around one-quarter of provincial spending on health care. In exchange, the provinces are expected to uphold five conditions: public administration, comprehensiveness, universality, portability, and accessibility.

The result of this federal legislation has been that all Canadian provinces and territories provide medically necessary care free at point of provision for hospital and physician services. But given the wide disparity in the size, demography, financial capacity, and political culture of Canadian provinces, notable differences in provincial health care exist.

Provinces are free to cover public services beyond hospital and physician care, if they can afford it; and even the interpretation of "medically necessary" can vary across provinces. Because of this, the level of public coverage for particular services, as well as the wait times for these services, can differ significantly from province to province. As this chapter describes, Nova Scotia's population exhibits some of the poorest health indicators across Canada. Unsurprisingly, it also has one of the oldest and poorest demographics in the country. Thus it must address the complex demands facing all modern health care systems, but with a more constrained financial base, an older and less healthy population, and a population size that precludes many economies of scale enjoyed by other provinces.

1.1 Geography and sociodemography

Given the status of Halifax as a major military and naval base from its founding in 1749, much of the social, political, and economic infrastructure of Nova Scotia has been shaped by its historical role. Because the health and well-being of military personnel in the eighteenth century were critical in protecting the colony from the French (until 1763) and then the Americans (until 1784), the early governors of Nova Scotia were quite aware of the need for effective and organized health care for their troops. Epidemics were important variables in eighteenth-century military planning, and key tactical manoeuvres (such as the British plan to place Louisbourg under siege in 1757, or the American plan to attack Halifax in 1775) were arguably called off because of the effect of smallpox outbreaks on military capacity (Marble, 1993). But the link between medical resources and military requirements was, in general, not a positive one for the colony as a whole. Medical supplies and personnel were largely limited to the military forces, and very few civilian doctors were available for the wider population. For much of the eighteenth century, hospital services for civilians were limited to those provided in the local poorhouse (Marble, 1993).

The tension between social and health policy was pronounced very early in Nova Scotia's history, as the need to support the destitute families of military personnel was cited as the reason that Halifax could not afford to develop suitable hospitals for its inhabitants. By the end of the eighteenth century, Nova Scotia's military role had declined as its importance as an immigration centre increased, but the tension between social and health care spending remained. Growing waves of Scottish and Irish emigration overwhelmed the province's capacity to deal with the large numbers of diseased and destitute immigrants arriving at the port, and one irate governor made a point of collecting poorhouse inhabitants in Halifax and sending them back to London (Marble, 1993).

In the nineteenth century, cholera and typhus replaced smallpox as the most feared diseases, and the conditions on ships transporting immigrants to Canada were so poor that the vessels became known as "coffin ships." Like Quebec, Nova Scotia was a key point of entry for new immigrants, and health care resources were focused on screening for, and circumscribing the spread of, virulent pathogens. Two hundred years later, chronic illnesses such as cancer and heart disease have replaced cholera and smallpox as major causes of mortality, and population outmigration has replaced immigration as a key policy concern. But Nova Scotia still remains economically dependent on the public sector (including the military), and it still must support a higher ratio of individuals with greater health care requirements compared to most other provinces.

The current population of Nova Scotia (943,002 in 2016) is, compared with much of Canada, quite homogeneous. The majority of the population has its roots in the waves of Anglo-Celtic migration, including not only British and Irish colonists but also the New England Planters and Loyalists who arrived from the south. While Nova Scotia is home to approximately 30,000 francophones, not all trace their ethnic origins to the Acadians, the descendants of the French settlers of the seventeenth and eighteenth centuries. There are also 20,790 Nova Scotians of African descent. Many are descended from those who migrated to Canada from the United States with the wave of Loyalists in the late 1700s and early 1800s. Approximately 33,950 individuals consider their ethnic origin to be First Nations, although only 12,910 have status under the Indian Act (and of these, 4,135 reside off reserve). Smaller numbers of visible minorities (mainly of African, Arab, Chinese, and South Asian descent) live predominantly in the Halifax Regional Municipality (Statistics Canada, 2011a & 2011b; Statistics Canada, 2016).

Of all the Canadian provinces, Nova Scotia spends the highest percentage of its budget on health care: 46 per cent, compared to the national average of 38 per cent (CIHI, 2015a, 17). A number of factors contribute to this trend. On the basis of population, Nova Scotia is the fourth-smallest province in Canada and it has the highest ratio in Canada of the population over 65 years of age, at 16.5 per cent (Statistics Canada, 2011c). For decades, the unemployment rate has remained consistently above the national average, and the direction of provincial mobility has

Figure 1.1 Map of Nova Scotia

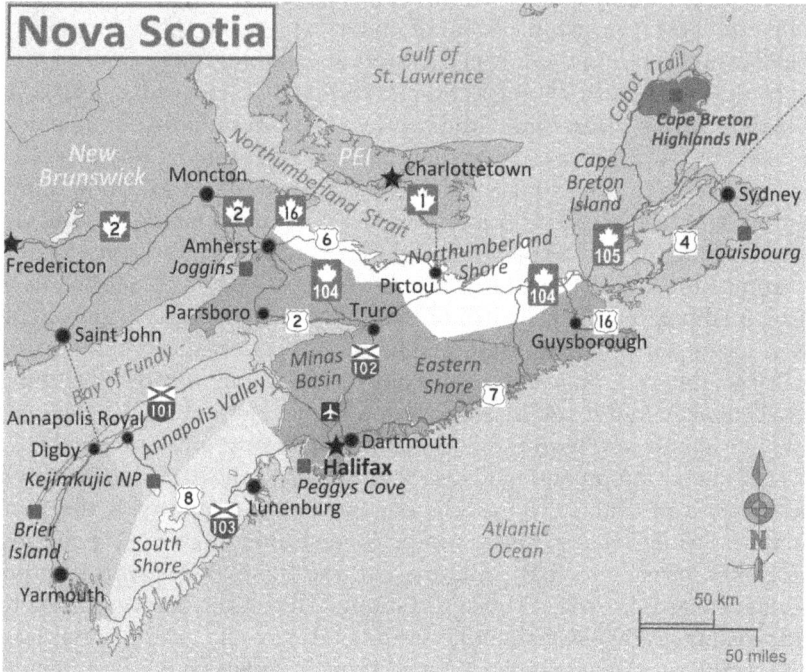

English map of Nova Scotia by Shaundd. Wikimedia Commons. Used under the CC BY-SA 3.0 licence.

generally been to outmigration, though the trend fluctuates from year to year. The vast majority of those leaving the province are between the ages of 20 and 34 (Employment and Development Canada, 2013). As in most provinces, there is a considerable urban-rural divide.

Figure 1.1 illustrates the regions and population centres of Nova Scotia, and Table 1.1 tracks population growth rates.

Geographically, the area around the Halifax Regional Municipality experiences the lowest utilization of Employment Insurance (1.5 per cent), with the rates increasing significantly the further one goes to the eastern or western peripheries (7.5 per cent on the eastern tip of Cape

Table 1.1 Main population centres with census growth rates, 1991–2011

	1991	1996	% change 1991–6	2001	% change 1996–2001	2006	% change 2001–6	2011	% change 2006–11
Nova Scotia	899,942	909,282	1.0	908,007	–0.1	913,462	0.6	921,727	0.9
Cape Breton*	–	117,849	–	109,330	–7.2	105,928	–3.1	101,619	–4.1
Halifax	330,979	342,966	3.6	359,183	4.7	372,858	3.8	390,328	4.7
Kentville	24,080	25,090	4.2	25,172	0.3	25,969	3.2	26,359	1.5
New Glasgow	38,664	38,055	–1.6	36,735	–3.5	36,288	–1.2	35,809	–1.3
Truro	42,697	44,102	3.3	44,276	0.4	45,077	1.8	45,888	1.8

*No data available for 1991
Source: Statistics Canada, Population and dwelling counts, 1996, 2001, 2006, and 2011.

Breton to the east, and 9.8 per cent in Shelburne County on the far western reaches of the province) (Nova Scotia Department of Finance, 2014a). With a population of almost 400,000, the Halifax Regional Municipality has just under half of the province's population. Yet the same region has only 12 of the province's 51 seats, which means that any government ignoring issues important to rural inhabitants does so at its peril. In a 2001 study of Canadian democratic representation, Donald Blake ranked Nova Scotia as the least democratic province due to its extreme disproportionality in voting power (Blake, 2001; see also Carbert, 2015).

1.2 Political context

Because of the province's relative cultural homogeneity and its large number of very long-standing communities, much literature has described the political culture of Nova Scotia as quite "traditional," with voting patterns based on historical family allegiances and a system of patronage politics forming the framework of policymaking (Beck, 1957). This perspective, identifying "localism, tradition, caution, stability, social order, hierarchical religions, and elitism in the economic and political realm" (Wiseman, 2007, 151) continues to inform some contemporary analyses of Maritime politics (see, e.g., Bricker & Ibbitson, 2013). However, as

Carbert (2015) argues, a more careful analysis shows that this model of politics is no more prevalent in Nova Scotia than in any other Canadian province. If there is a distinctive historical legacy in Nova Scotia's political culture, she concludes, "it may be the high culture of public administration that congealed when Halifax was established as an outpost of the British Empire" (p. 14).

To a considerable degree, the current political discourse in Nova Scotia is focused on the tension between the creation of jobs and the need to increase employment on the one hand and the need to contain public spending and lower public debt on the other. This creates serious friction in debates over health care policy. While the health care sector in general, and health care workers in particular, are seen as serious cost drivers in an already-expensive system, the health care sector is also the source of a large number of (often well-paying and secure) jobs: in 2012, approximately 69,000 individuals were employed within the health care and social assistance sector (Employment and Development Canada, 2012). There has in consequence been little political motivation, despite rhetoric, to reduce health spending by reducing the number of health care workers. Rather, the political focus has increasingly been on the wage levels and remuneration of health care professionals.

Due in part both to Nova Scotia's relatively small size and to the long-standing relationship between the political and medical elites in the province, the relationship between physicians and policymakers has historically been relatively close and remarkably opaque. In contrast to the acrimonious public skirmishes between the provincial government and nurses, home health care workers, and paramedics, the province has generally been willing to accommodate the policy concerns of physicians (Boase, 1994). As Bickerton notes, "Nova Scotia was one of the most traditional of provinces in its approach to the health care system. The province and its physicians had an unbroken record of harmonious negotiation over fee schedules ... There was not any predilection on the part of the province to question or challenge the physician-dominated, hierarchical model of health care" (1999, 166). The one remarkable exception to this was the 1993–7 Liberal government of Premier John Savage. Savage was a well-respected medical doctor, and he appointed another well-regarded physician, Ron Stewart, as minister of health. Because of their clear understanding of the province's health care system, the Savage government presented a profound set of reforms to the organization of provincial health care administration (see chapter 2). Yet even they did not appreciate the established power of the provincial physicians' association, and an attempt to cut doctors' fees resulted in a large advertising campaign by the Nova Scotia Medical Society attacking both the premier and the health minister (MacLeod, 2006, 566). Relations between the government and physicians became fractious once again in 2015, when the Liberal government entered into salary negotiations with a focus on curtailing public spending. In the end, however, the physicians' contract dispute was resolved more expeditiously than those with other health care groups (see chapter 7).

With a population 14 times smaller than that of Ontario (and with less than a quarter of the population of provinces such as British Columbia or Alberta), Nova Scotia has little political influence at the federal level. In 1870 Nova Scotia had 21 of the House of Commons' 180 seats (11.66 per cent of the seats). Given the recent expansion of seats in the House of Commons due to western population growth, Nova Scotia now has only 11 out of 338 seats (3.25 per cent), a clear empirical marker of its loss of influence on the national stage. Politically, this means that it has little voice when confronted with national policies and strategies (such as the 2011 funding formula for the Canada Health Transfer) that disadvantaged provinces with weaker economies and older populations.

1.3 Economic context

The economy of nineteenth-century Nova Scotia was based largely on staple production (predominantly the fishery and forestry), but preferential trading ties with Great Britain, along with reciprocity agreements with the United States, facilitated the development of a strong mercantile trade. Nova Scotia's shipbuilding industry was a major part of this economy. Following Confederation in 1867 and the implementation of Canada's National Policy in 1879, however, the lucrative north-south trade patterns shifted to east-west routes following the St. Lawrence River. Increasing population density in Central Canada meant larger markets, which shifted the pools of investment capital away from the Atlantic region. Given competition from the industrial heartland, along with high transportation costs, Nova Scotia's manufacturing sector (producing goods such as textiles and furniture, along with iron and steel production) sharply diminished in the first half of the twentieth century (Nova Scotia, 2014a; Carbert, 2015).

By the middle of the twentieth century, the province's economy had stabilized somewhat due to the introduction of federal programs such as unemployment insurance, federal equalization, the public pension plan, public health care, and the Canada Assistance Program. Federal and provincial governments jointly funded regional development programs and public enterprises such as the Cape Breton Development Corporation (DEVCO) and Sydney Steel (SYSCO). But by the 1980s, the public sector (federal and provincial) in Nova Scotia was responsible for more than 40 per cent of the province's GDP. This was the highest level of any Canadian province (Nova Scotia, 2014a, 14).

Beginning in the early 1990s, the economic environment worsened sharply. In 1992 the federal government closed the cod fishery, a staple of the fishing sector. In the same year offshore oil and gas production began, but it was never to be as lucrative as Newfoundland's offshore industry. One of the few remaining coal mines in the province closed in 1992 after a serious underground explosion killed all 26 miners working at the time, and the last coal mine in Cape Breton closed in 2001. This was the same year that the Sydney Steel Corporation shut down its steel production. Two large military bases (Cornwallis and Shearwater) were closed in the mid-1990s. Even the forestry sector was hit quite hard when two of the province's major pulp and paper mills closed in 2012. Nova Scotia does have a small manufacturing sector, but it constitutes only 1.76 per cent of all Canadian manufacturing sales (Nova Scotia Department of Finance, 2013).

It is not surprising, then, that Nova Scotia relies so heavily on federal transfers. In 2016–17, the province received just over three billion dollars from Ottawa. Of this, $943 million was directed through the Canada Health Transfer, $349 million was allocated through the Canada Social Transfer, $1.72 billion came in the form of equalization payments, and $49 million was allotted through the 2005 offshore accord (Finance Canada, 2016). Nova Scotia's gross net debt by 2013 was $16.4 billion, an increase of more than 13 per cent ($1.6 billion) over the previous 10 years. Net debt per capita in 2013 amounted to $14,832. Net debt as a percentage of total revenue by 2013 was 138.1 per cent (36.7 per cent of provincial GDP); while debt servicing costs in Nova Scotia by the end of fiscal year 2013 were $921 million, which amounted to 9.1 per cent of total revenues (Nova Scotia Office of the Auditor General, 2014a, chapter 4). Over the period 1990 to 2009, Nova Scotia's rate of economic growth (measured in total growth in real GDP) was, at 40.6 per cent, lower than every other Canadian province and 7.2 per cent lower than the national average (see Figure 1.2).

Nova Scotia's working-age population is forecast to decline by 20 per cent in 2036, with a loss of approximately 100,000 individuals between the ages of 18 and 65 (Nova Scotia, 2014a, 12). This decrease is not balanced

Figure 1.2 Total economic growth in real GDP, 1990–2009

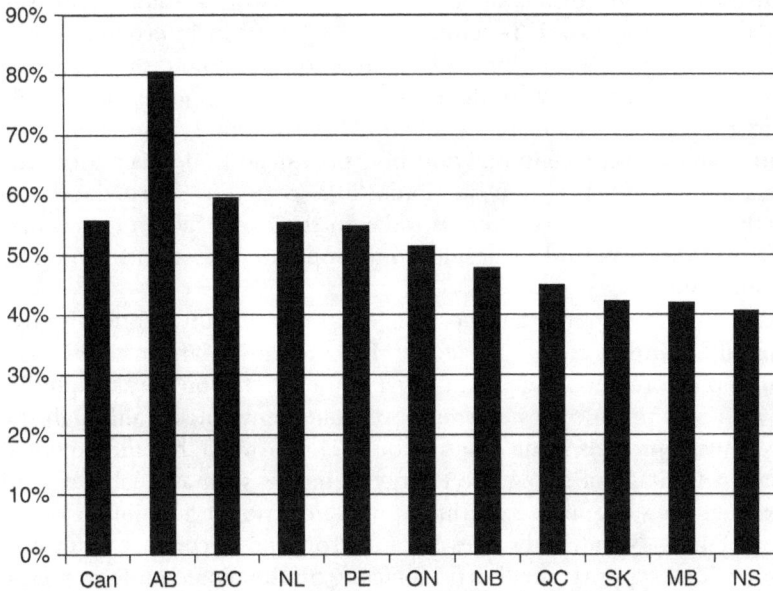

Source: *The Report of the Nova Scotia Commission on Building Our New Economy*, February 2014, p. 16.

by immigration, as the province's immigration rate is 3.3 times lower than the Canadian average (ibid., 25). Added to the problem of a decreasing labour force is the ongoing issue of weak private-sector capital formation that has confounded the Nova Scotia economy for well over a century. Despite public attempts to support credit and equity investments, average annual per-capita venture capital investment remains lower than the national average, and considerably lower than that in Quebec, British Columbia, and Ontario (although, interestingly, it is higher than that in Manitoba, Saskatchewan, and Alberta: see Nova Scotia, 2014a, 21). Most businesses in Nova Scotia are very small: the majority of manufacturing enterprises in the province, for example, have fewer than 20 employees; a scant 7.2 per cent have more than 20 (ibid., 187). One reason for the tension between small businesses (often referred to as the "backbone of the economy") and large ones is that considerably more employment is generated by big business. 62 per cent of Nova Scotia's businesses employ fewer than five people, yet these same businesses employ only 8 per cent of the province's total employees. Conversely, only 2 per cent of businesses in the province have more than 500 employees, yet these industries account for *half* of all provincial employees (ibid., 32). Given that the greatest growth potential is to be found in international and interprovincial trade, the province is at a considerable disadvantage as smaller firms find it more difficult to seek out trade opportunities. While trade growth for Canada as a whole in 2012 was only 1.5 per cent, Nova Scotia's share of international and interprovincial trade decreased dramatically over the past decade (ibid., 29): "Stated as sharply and succinctly as possible, Nova Scotia is today in the early stages of what may be a prolonged period of accelerating population loss and economic decline" (ibid., 4).

There are some potentially positive features within this economic environment. Planned energy projects (Muskrat Falls, Maritime Link, and various offshore developments) as well as the $25 billion naval shipbuilding plan may provide jobs and support related enterprises, although the fate of these projects is uncertain at best. The province has the potential to take advantage of renewable energy resources such as tidal and wind power, and has begun to experiment with tidal power generation in the Bay of Fundy. Nova Scotia does have a strong postsecondary education sector, which supports small firms focusing on the biotechnology, health care, information technology, pharmaceutical, digital media, aerospace, and defence sectors. The workforce, compared to the national average, contains a high proportion of individuals with trade certifications or university/college degrees. Nonetheless, governments have very little room for fiscal manoeuvre; most public spending is already accounted for, and new programs require politically unattractive measures such as new taxation, cuts to existing programs, or deficit financing. In smaller jurisdictions, the ability for a government to make substantial changes to a province's economic trajectory is even more limited. As a former Nova Scotia finance minister pointed out, "Nova Scotia is a tiny piece of the continental and global economy with limited natural resources and a dependence on imported fossil fuels for energy. A small change in interest rates or the U.S. dollar exchange rate has more impact on the Nova Scotia economy than every combined tool available to the provincial government" (Steele, 2014a, 162).

1.4 Health status of the population

Until 1991, the median age in Nova Scotia remained under the Canadian average. But throughout the 1990s, the province experienced a

Table 1.2 Median population age, 1921–2011

	1921	1931	1941	1951	1961	1971	1981	1991	2001	2011
Canada	23.9	24.7	27.0	27.7	26.3	26.2	29.6	33.5	37.6	40.6
NS	23.6	24.1	25.8	26.5	24.9	25.4	29.3	33.4	38.8	43.7

Source: Statistics Canada, http://www12.statcan.gc.ca/census-recensement/2011/as-sa/fogs-spg/Facts-pr-eng.cfm?Lang=Eng&GC=12

net population outmigration as working-age individuals moved west in search of employment. By 2011, the difference between the provincial and national median age was a striking 3.1 years (Table 1.2).

By 2011, 16.6 per cent of Nova Scotia's population was over the age of 65 (Statistics Canada, 2011d). This is projected to increase to at least 28.4 per cent by 2031 (Nova Scotia Health Research Foundation, 2009). Simply stated, Nova Scotia has a higher proportion of individuals over 65 compared to all other provinces and territories (although the ratio in New Brunswick is very close), a demographic that utilizes a higher proportion of health care services. At the same time, the province is experiencing a net outflow of individuals who use proportionally fewer health services and who are net contributors to the tax base. Given the province's older demographic, Nova Scotia has higher rates of arthritis, diabetes, high blood pressure, chronic obstructive pulmonary disease, heart attack, and stroke than the country as a whole (Statistics Canada, 2013). Sixty-one per cent of Nova Scotians are overweight or obese (compared to the national average of 52 per cent); 22 per cent are smokers (20 per cent across Canada); 28 per cent are heavy drinkers (24 per cent across Canada); and 34 per cent consume fruits and vegetables five or more times per day (40 per cent across Canada). The incidence of new cases of cancer is 423 per 100,000 Nova Scotians, compared to 391 per 100,000 Canadians (Nova Scotia Department of Health and Wellness, 2015a). Certain indicators of poor health, such as arthritis and heart disease, might be explained statistically because of the province's higher proportion of older adults. However, Nova Scotia also scores poorly in other health indicators in which it is less clear that age is an explanatory variable. In 2012, for example, 32 per cent of Nova Scotians between the ages of 12 and 17 reported being overweight or obese, compared to the national average of 21.8 per cent, while 51.9 per cent of Nova Scotians between the ages of 20 and 34 reported being overweight or obese (compared to 41.1 per cent nationally). In 2013, 33.5 per cent of those 20 to 34 years of age in Nova Scotia consumed the recommended daily servings of fruits and vegetables, compared to the national average of 42.3 per cent (Community Foundations of Nova Scotia, 2011). According to the 2013 Canadian Tobacco, Alcohol and Drugs Survey, Nova Scotia's smoking rate increased even as the national rate decreased. Broken down by age, 21 per cent of those in the 20-to-24-year-old group were smokers, and 27.1 per cent of those in the 25-to-44-year-old range were smokers, compared to only 16.4 per cent of those over 45 (Canada, 2013).

Perceived mental health in Nova Scotia is very similar to the national average (71.8 per cent to 72.2 per cent respectively reporting very good or excellent mental health). But life satisfaction in Nova Scotia is slightly higher than the national average, while perceived life stress is discernibly lower. Suicide rates are lower in Nova Scotia (9.1 per 100,000) compared to the national rate (10.2 per 100,000). Rates of hospitalization due to mental illness (per 100,000) are lower than the national average (401 for Nova Scotia, 489 for Canada), while mental illness inpatient days (per 10,000) are considerably lower (581 for Nova Scotia and 707 for Canada). The rate for repeat hospitalization for mental illness in Nova Scotia is 9.6 per cent, compared to the national average 10.9 per cent (Statistics Canada, 2013). Treatment rates, however, are an inconclusive measure of mental health, as lower rates could either indicate lower rates of illness, on the one hand, or insufficient resources for treatment, on the other.

An even more equivocal pattern exists for children and youth in Nova Scotia. In 2013, 98.0 per cent of 12- to 19-year-olds in Nova Scotia reported being satisfied or very satisfied with their lives (the highest among all provinces and higher than the national average of 96.3 per cent). A major depressive episode was experienced by 8.3 per cent of Nova Scotian youths aged 15 to 24 in 2012, compared to 10.7 per cent nationally. However, in the same year, 9.8 per cent of Nova Scotian youths aged 15 to 24 thought about taking their lives over a 12-month period, a figure that was 69 per cent higher than the national average and the highest among all provinces. Similarly, Nova Scotia's rate of anxiety disorder for youth aged 15 to 24 years, at 10.2 per cent, is considerably higher than the national rate of 6.3 per cent (Community Foundations of Nova Scotia, 2014a).

1.5 Summary

Chronic diseases in Nova Scotia tend to be higher overall than the national average, accounting for more than 70 per cent of the economic burden of illness in the province (Nova Scotia Health Research Foundation,

2009). This can partially be explained by the larger number of older individuals in the province. However, risk factors for poor health, including obesity, nutrition, smoking, and mental health issues were also more pronounced in children and youth in the province. There is some debate about the degree to which poorer levels of health in the province are a consequence of relative income disparities independent of age. One study, for example, notes that Nova Scotia has the highest percentage of households experiencing food insecurity (14.6 per cent) and argues that improving the incomes of those at the bottom of the income scale could improve health outcomes (cited in Nova Scotia Health Research Foundation, 2009). The province has recognized that regardless of age, the major chronic diseases are influenced by modifiable risk factors, and some programs have been developed to address them.

Nonetheless, the outlook for the province is challenging. Like other Maritime provinces, the labour force is diminishing, productivity growth is poor, and job-growth performance is stagnant. The proportion of Nova Scotians above the age of 65 continues to increase, which not only removes taxable income from the economy but also increases the amount of public spending on health care. And while there is some debate about whether the health care cost equated with seniors' care in the future will or will not rise dramatically due to the improving health status of those over 65, this benefit will be unlikely in Nova Scotia given the relatively poor general health indicators for all ages compared to the rest of Canada. In addition, given the combination of demographic challenges and marginal economic performance, overall prospects relative to the rest of Canada are poor. Saillant (2016) argues that while provinces such as British Columbia and Ontario may be able to withstand the shock of population aging, health care in the Atlantic provinces is "simply not sustainable without massive amounts of new funding from Ottawa" (94). Although the smaller and faster-aging populations will feel the effects of these economic and demographic trends most keenly, these socioeconomic shifts will also present real challenges to the political dynamics of federal governance in Canada.

Chapter Two

Organization and Regulation

The key to understanding health care as a *system* is to identify how decision-making authority is structured. This authority can be delegated to many different agents, including regulated health care professionals, regional administrative units, or discrete private for-profit or not-for-profit bodies. This chapter begins by situating discussions of governance mechanisms within a historical context. As Marmor and Wendt (2012) note, historical legacies can be quite important in understanding health policy development. The provision of health care in eighteenth- and nineteenth-century Nova Scotia was, as it was in the rest of Canada, predominantly a "local and private" matter, and the 1867 Constitution Act determined it to be a provincial responsibility precisely for that reason. But the growing cost and complexity of health care led to a major change in the way that these services were provided across Canada. With the passage of the 1957 federal Hospital Insurance and Diagnostic Services Act and the 1966 Medical Care Act, Ottawa persuaded the provinces to provide universal public insurance to their respective populations by promising dollar-for-dollar reimbursement for physician and hospital services. In Nova Scotia, the development of a public insurance system was closely tied to the existing private not-for-profit insurance program run by the physicians' association, so much so that the private agency administering the existing private insurance system was given a special "public" status in order to remain the body overseeing the new public program.

Following the establishment of the public insurance system, the most consequential governance debate has focused on the optimal degree of authority to be distributed within provinces on a geographical basis. The implementation of public insurance in each province had resulted in an "agency" model of health care governance (Tuohy, 2003), in which departments of health delegated to health care providers the responsibility to use public health care funds in an appropriate way (i.e., for "medically necessary" care). But physicians had no direct incentive to ration health care resources, and cost and coordination issues led provincial governments to consider the need to reassert more control over the provision of health care. The rise of New Public Management theory, with its twin themes of accountability and devolved responsibility, promised both cost control and user responsiveness (Aucoin, 1995). But one key aspect of New Public Management, the privatization of services, was not deemed politically viable for Canadian health care; and the operationalization of New Public Management principles in health care systems was largely limited to the implementation of regionalized administrative structures. (For a more detailed discussion of New Public Management principles in Canadian health care, see Fierlbeck, 2011.)

There is no clear definition of "regionalization" (as distinct, e.g., from devolution or decentralization [Lomas, 1996]), although Lewis and Kouri (2004, 14) see regionalization in Canada as characterized by defined geography, devolved authority, consolidated municipal authority, and responsibility for a range of health services. Between 1992 and 1997, nine provinces and territories introduced a system of regional health authorities (RHAs). Quebec had already implemented them in 1989; while Ontario established local health integration networks in 2006 (Marchildon, 2016). The stated objectives of regionalized health care were quite varied, ranging from the integration of similar services or institutions (such as small hospitals); the integration of different kinds of services (e.g., making psychological counselling more readily accessible to cancer patients); the adoption of evidence-based practice; the identification of particular needs in specific populations; public engagement; and increased accountability (Marchildon, 2016). While not explicitly stated, another goal was to counterbalance or destabilize entrenched health care interest groups such as professional associations, health care unions, and some large institutions (Denis, Contandriopoulos, & Beaulieu, 2004; Black & Fierlbeck, 2006; Fierlbeck, 2016).

But as this chapter describes, Nova Scotia has recently joined those provinces amalgamating their RHAs into a single entity. Again, situating the discussion of regionalization within a historical context is informative, as the narrative justifying the establishment, expansion, and amalgamation of RHAs shows an interesting pattern: regardless of whether the government of the day chose to expand or contract the number of regions, the broad justifications offered for the restructuring (greater efficiency, accountability, and responsiveness) have remained the same. The narrative underlying the amalgamation of RHAs to a single body in 2015 was that the province's Department of Health and Wellness (DHW) was to focus on planning and priorities, while the Nova Scotia Health Authority was to manage the day-to-day operations. This account is precisely the same one given for the implementation of a more *regionalized* structure in 1996. Despite the number of health authorities, however, certain governance issues remain constant. As Lewis and Kouri (2004, 27) suggest, for example, governments can have a hard time deciding "whether they can and should get out of the management business"; and confusion (or tension) regarding the appropriate division of activity by health authorities and departments of health remains a feature of provinces adopting a single health authority structure, just as it was for those with several RHAs. A more detailed analysis of what the consolidated Nova Scotia Health Authority can hope to achieve, as well as some of the potential pitfalls it may encounter, will be presented in chapter 8.

2.1 Overview and history

Halifax's early reputation was of "a port of disease and pestilence" (Marble, 2006, 139). This is perhaps unsurprising, given its position at the entrance of a large natural harbour. Acting as a centre for international commercial trade and the transfer of troops and prisoners of war, as well as a port of entry for immigrants, the city experienced notable epidemics of smallpox, cholera, and typhus fever, which shaped the development of the province's health care system. Yet it is also interesting to note that the leading cause of death in the first half of the nineteenth century was not disease, but accidents (Table 2.1). Between 1800 and 1850, a third of all deaths in Nova Scotia could be attributed to unintentional injury, while all communicable diseases combined contributed another third. By 2009, cancer and heart disease accounted for half of all deaths in the province, while less than 3 per cent of deaths were due to a communicable disease (mostly influenza).

Nova Scotia's strategic geopolitical relevance in the eighteenth century was, at best, an ambivalent variable in the historical development of its health care system. Despite the large numbers of highly qualified medical personnel who arrived in Nova Scotia to tend to the health of the military troops (340 surgeons alone between 1749 and 99), the British did not assume responsibility for the health of their colonists through either the provision of competent medical professionals or the building

Table 2.1 Causes of death, Nova Scotia, 1800–50 and 2009

1800–50	%	2009	%
Accidents	35.6	Cancer	30.0
Smallpox	16.3	Heart disease	20.4
Consumption (TB)	8.2	Stroke	6.2
Cholera	5.5	Respiratory disease	5.5
Neuropathy	4.7	Unintentional injuries	5.3
Scarlet fever	4.4	Alzheimer's	3.3
Violence	4.3	Diabetes	2.7
Respiratory diseases	3.9	Influenza and pneumonia	2.2

Sources: Marble, 2006, 175; Statistics Canada, Leading Causes of Death in Canada, 2009, available at http://www.statcan.gc.ca/pub/84-215-x/2012001/tbl/T016-eng.pdf.

of hospitals (Marble, 1993, 3, 26, 185). For more than a hundred years, the only hospital accessible to the public was to be found in the local poorhouse (there were, however, discrete hospitals for the Navy, Army, mariners, and prisoners of war). Just as today, health policy in the eighteenth and nineteenth centuries was often shaped as a response to serious public health crises. No public health officer, for example, was appointed to inspect immigrant ships for smallpox or typhus fever until 1827, when a serious epidemic precipitated the appointment of the position (though it is also unclear how difficult it was to fill the position, given the statistically high likelihood that the recipient would perish from the very diseases he was expected to control: see Marble, 2006).

Then as now, as well, the development of health infrastructure was hobbled by the political division between rural and urban constituencies. Halifax, with the largest port, experienced the highest occurrence of disease; but it had already committed financially to the development of municipal services such as fire protection, water supply, sewage, street lighting, and city prisons and could not on its own afford the considerable costs of establishing a general public hospital as well. The House of Assembly in Nova Scotia was in a far better position to raise these funds; but as only a minority of the seats were held by representatives from Halifax, attempts to establish a hospital in Halifax were challenged by those who felt that they would be taxed to provide a service they would be highly unlikely to use (Marble, 2006). Finally, with a limited grant from the province, as well as private funding, the first designated general hospital in the province, the City and Provincial Hospital, opened to the public in the 1860s.

Private subscriptions and earmarked levies were a common method of financing large capital projects in the nineteenth century. During the War of 1812, for example, the considerable sum of 10,000 pounds had been collected by the British military through a port tax in eastern Maine (the Castine Funds). While there had been some expectation that these funds would be used to establish a new alms house in the province, the Earl of Dalhousie, governor of Nova Scotia, decided instead to use the funds to establish a "college of learning." It was some time before this institution included a faculty of medicine, however, largely because there was no public general hospital available for the training of resident physicians. Once this barrier was overcome, the attempt to set up a faculty for the instruction of medical doctors was then obstructed by the fact that the practice of dissection was still illegal within the province (but given the significant proportion of doctors sitting in the House of Assembly, this obstacle was quickly eliminated). Within a few years of Confederation, Halifax could finally boast of a large public hospital, a faculty of medicine, and a modern psychiatric hospital (Marble, 2006).

When it opened, the City and Provincial Hospital provided 50 beds. By 1892, the now renamed Victoria General Hospital had 180 beds, which expanded to 250 beds in 1922 and 400 beds in 1948 (Nova Scotia, 1950, 3). In contrast, the current Queen Elizabeth II Health Sciences Centre has a capacity of 1,380 beds, with outpatient visits numbering approximately 739,286 per year (Capital District Health Authority [CDHA], 2013). For much of the nineteenth and twentieth centuries, the city of Halifax was informally segregated between Protestant and Roman Catholic institutions, including schools, universities, and sports and leisure facilities. Hospitals were no different, and until 1973 the Halifax Infirmary (founded by the Sisters of Charity of St. Vincent de Paul in 1886) served unofficially as the Roman Catholic hospital. The infirmary was then taken over by the province and merged with the federally run veterans' hospital (Camp Hill) in 1988. Between 1994 and 1996, the Victoria General, the Halifax Infirmary, the Camp Hill Hospital, and the Abbie Lane Hospital were formally merged into the present Queen Elizabeth II Health Sciences Centre.

Hospitals began to be established in the surrounding communities within a few decades of the founding of the City and Provincial Hospital. Springhill opened a hospital in 1893, as did New Glasgow in 1895. Eight more were opened throughout the province in the first decade of the twentieth century. In 1949, Nova Scotia (like many other provinces) received a Federal Health Survey Grant to take stock of the province's health care infrastructure. This followed the 1945 and 1946 Dominion-Provincial first ministers' conferences on postwar reconstruction, at

Table 2.2 Inventory of hospitals in Nova Scotia, 1949

Type	Number	Notes
General	10	Bed capacity < 20
	16	Bed capacity 20–49
	5	Bed capacity 50–99
	6	Bed capacity 100+
	7	Under construction
Pediatric	1	
Maternity	3	
Infectious	1	
TB	4	Does not include 2 annexed to other hospitals
Mental	19	
Veterans'	1	
Defence	1	
Total	**74**	

Source: Nova Scotia, *Report on the Survey of Hospitals in Nova Scotia under the Federal Health Survey Grant, 1949.* Halifax, 1950.

which the possibility of a federal hospital insurance system was broached. In anticipation that demands for hospital care would increase significantly were a compulsory hospital-insurance system to be introduced, Ottawa encouraged the provinces to take inventory of what services existed, the rate of utilization of such services, and any notable gaps or deficiencies in care. From the resulting health survey report, we have a remarkably clear picture of what Nova Scotia's health system looked like in 1949.

By 1949, Nova Scotia could boast of 66 hospitals, with several more under construction (Table 2.2). The average hospital stay in 1948 lasted 7.3 days, with 13 per cent of the total population having been hospitalized (Nova Scotia, 1950, 31, 133). No doubt the rising number of hospital births contributed to the latter figure: in 1925, only 10.5 per cent of all live births occurred in a hospital setting, compared to 79.6 per cent in 1948 (31). Costs per patient-day rose from $2.67 in 1935 to $7.67 in 1948, an increase of 187.2 per cent (73). Hospitals consumed 13 per cent of total expenditure for health services, while physicians accounted for 39.8 per cent, and drugs for 12.9 per cent (110). In 2014, in contrast, hospitals accounted for 30 per cent of the province's health care budget, physicians 15 per cent, and drugs 16 per cent (CIHI, 2014). Just under 20 per cent of the population in 1949 held private (Blue Cross) health insurance (Nova Scotia, 1950, 102), which had been introduced into the Maritimes in 1943. Two of the hospitals were owned by the Nova Scotia government (the only province in addition to Newfoundland, noted the health survey report, "in which general hospitals are owned and operated by the provincial government" [3]). Eighteen hospitals were owned by voluntary community organizations, eight by local governments, nine by church organizations, and three by associations of industrial workers (119).

Many of the concerns highlighted by the 1950 health survey report seem remarkably prescient. Even in 1949 apprehension was being expressed over the high costs of inpatient care, and much of this was in turn related to the rise in the number of chronically ill patients (though the most common chronic disease of this period was tuberculosis rather than cancer, diabetes, or heart disease). Consequently, the report stressed the need to develop preventive health care and establish a larger number of nursing homes for the treatment of the chronically ill. Other recommendations with a palpably modern sensibility include the call to establish group practices and the suggestion that the management of hospitals and hospital planning should be more integrated at the provincial level. The last point illustrates how health care since the founding of Halifax in 1749 to the late 1940s had been very organic: it was developed when and where it was needed (albeit at times after a great deal of effort), and it was largely financed and run at a local level. "Although comments are sometimes made concerning the 'Hospital system' of Nova Scotia," notes the health survey report, "no such system exists. There is no organization or integration either on a provincial or regional basis. Communities, large and small, have been provided with hospital services by the efforts of various individuals or groups without any definite plan or over-all system" (Nova Scotia, 1950, 147). The idea that provincial health care was a *systemic* entity, and that the provincial government had a role to play in shaping it, began to inform Nova Scotia policymaking only in the last half of the twentieth century.

As in most provinces, the move to thinking about an integrated provincial health care *system* began with the discussion over public health coverage. Compulsory health insurance itself was not a new concept in Nova Scotia, which likely enjoyed the first comprehensive medical-coverage program in Canada. The "check-off" health insurance system implemented by Cape Breton coal companies in the mid to late nineteenth century was a mandatory condition of employment in which weekly pay deductions entitled miners and their dependents to "unlimited physician visits, a range of medications, surgical procedures, and hospital services" (McAlister & Twohig, 2005, 1504). Services and fees were negotiated by the coal company, the union, and the physicians, and lasted until the implementation of public insurance for medical services in Nova Scotia. Another early example of health insurance in Nova Scotia dates back to 1782: workers labouring in the Naval Dockyards could, with a deduction of four pence per month, expect medical assistance, such as it was, should they require it (Marble, 1993, 131).

But universal hospital coverage was a new phenomenon. The debate over the introduction of publicly insured hospital insurance in 1959 was relatively muted in Nova Scotia, compared to the more acrimonious discussion in many other provinces. This was likely due to the timing of the legislation, as Nova Scotia introduced its public hospital insurance plan 2 years after federal legislation, and at least a year after Saskatchewan, Manitoba, Alberta, British Columbia, and Newfoundland introduced provincial public insurance plans. The Nova Scotia Medical Society was keenly aware that the plan had not only been endorsed by the Canadian Medical Society but had also been sanctioned by "the results of the recent Saskatchewan election." The society was thus guardedly conciliatory over the introduction of public hospital insurance, and it asserted to its members that "given the whole-hearted support of their profession, The Medical Society of Nova Scotia can succeed in retaining in this province a large measure of the traditional ideals and freedoms of practice within the framework of a comprehensive medical service available to all who wish to participate" (Nova Scotia Medical Society, 1960, 1). The society was widely consulted in developing the legislation, and its views were very evident in the Nova Scotia Hospitals Act and its supporting regulations.

Ten years later, Nova Scotia introduced its public insurance program for physician services. The administrative development of this program was considerably easier than the hospital insurance program had been, as the province already had a voluntary prepaid nonprofit plan for medical services. Sponsored by the Medical Society of Nova Scotia, the Maritime Medical Care Plan had been established in 1948. Within 10 years, the Maritime Medical Care Plan had approximately 130,000 subscribers. The plan was affiliated with the Trans Canada Medical Plan overseen by the Canadian Medical Association, which attempted (with some difficulty) to coordinate health insurance across many Canadian provinces (Fraser, 1961). In 1960, Maritime Medical Care introduced the first health insurance plan in Canada designed specifically for the elderly. Because the Maritime Medical Care Plan was largely controlled by physicians, there was some resistance on the part of the Medical Society to a compulsory public plan. In 1963, the Medical Society presented a plan for coverage for the whole population; this plan was essentially a system of voluntary subscription to "approved carriers" by those who could afford them, and subsidies to those who could not. This idea was quickly overshadowed by the 1964 Hall Commission Report, which instead recommended a universal and compulsory approach to health coverage. Given that only 40 per cent of Nova Scotians had private health insurance at this time (Bickerton, 1999, 166), and given the dollar-for-dollar cost-sharing proposal of federal legislation introduced in 1966, the advantage of a government-sponsored plan was quite clear. On 1 April 1968, Maritime Medical Care began to administer the new Medical Services Insurance (MSI) plan.

The role of Maritime Medical Care in the development of Nova Scotia's public health care system is quite remarkable. From the beginning, the province strongly favoured the involvement of Maritime Medical Care in running a government-sponsored plan due to its administrative and actuarial expertise and because of the excellent relationship Maritime Medical Care had with Nova Scotia physicians. Given the short time frame set out by Ottawa for the development of medical insurance, provincial officials were dubious that the province would have enough expertise and resources to develop a viable plan de novo. Federal officials were sympathetic to the proposal to use the privately held Maritime Medical Care but felt that the stipulation of "public administration" in the federal medicare legislation under section 4(1)(a) precluded a doctor-sponsored plan. The door opened a crack in 1965 when Judy LaMarsh, federal minister of Health and Welfare, was reported to have stated that she would not rule out the possibility of a province developing a "two-tier" system in which a doctor-sponsored plan acted "in certain respects" as a province's agent (Nova Scotia, 1967, 137). This was possibly due to the fact that Saskatchewan's medicare system already had two doctor-sponsored plans operating concurrently with the new public plan, albeit only as "post offices" that received claims from doctors and forwarded them to the province's Medical Care Insurance Advisory Commission (or received cheques from the Commission and mailed them to doctors). Nova Scotia officials appealed to incoming federal minister of Health and Welfare Allan MacEachen, whose federal constituency happened to be in Cape Breton. MacEachen responded that Maritime Medical Care could be used to the extent desired, if provincial legislation were altered to assign to Maritime Medical Care "as part of the provincial authority" the role of assessing and approving accounts. In effect, the corporate status of Maritime Medical Care would have to be altered "to have one company represent the private side and another to represent the public side" (Nova Scotia, 1967, 145). Much negotiation ensued regarding the particular nature of this legislation, as Ottawa was quite concerned that the outcome would have "far reaching implications with regard to the establishment of the public authority in other provinces" (ibid., 141). In the end, Ottawa eventually accepted the concept of two separate entities within a single insurance authority. The public side of Maritime Medical Care became answerable to the minister of health, while the private side did not. The result of this curious legacy is that a significant component of Nova Scotia's current health care system is administered by a large private nonprofit organization that not only executes a number of major public functions but also owns and operates several private for-profit health care companies (see section 2.2.3).

One year following the implementation of the Medical Care Insurance Act, the province established the Nova Scotia Council of Health to advise on health service planning and utilization. The first major document produced by the council was *Health Care in Nova Scotia: A New Direction for the Seventies* (1972) and, in contrast to the guarded optimism of the public insurance advisory commission reports, the tone of *A New Direction for the Seventies* was almost apocalyptic. Warning of "the approaching crisis," the report began by stating that "increasing demands arising from the introduction of hospital and medical insurance have placed the quality of the entire health system in jeopardy" (Nova Scotia, 1972, i). Given the financial statistics presented in the report, there was clear justification for the alarm. The average escalation rate in health care spending between 1966 and 1972 was 12.5 per cent. Overall health costs in the province in 1960 amounted to $49,253,000. By 1965 this had increased to $78,439,000; and in 5 years this amount had almost doubled again to $140,653,000 (ibid., 4, 7). The report identifies three reasons for this escalation:

- increased use of the system through public response to opportunities created by hospital and medical insurance;
- the growing use of the most highly trained technical personnel in hospitals to provide all services, regardless of the skills required; and
- increases in salaries and wages. (Nova Scotia, 1972, 5)

What is remarkable in this report is the modern-sounding analysis not only of the systemic problems of health care delivery but also of the strategies for dealing with them. In addition to moving away from hospital-based treatments (as hospitals accounted for two-thirds of health care spending), the report called for administrative integration, a more effective utilization of health care personnel, more emphasis on disease prevention, and improved evaluative standards and assessment methods.

The 1972 report was the first attempt to superimpose a rationalized, overarching structure on Nova Scotia's health care system. The report approvingly cited England's 1972 White Paper on NHS Reorganization, which stated that "[a]dministrative reorganization within a unified health service that is closely linked with parallel local government services will provide a sure foundation for better services for all" (Nova Scotia, 1972, 27). The Council of Health sketched out a system of community health boards at the local level that would be responsible to a smaller number of regional health boards, which themselves would answer to a single provincial health commission. The health commission would be responsible to the minister of health for the overall planning and implementation of health services. A second major report on health-professions licensing was commissioned in 1974, and it was presented in 1976. As Boase notes, regulation of the health professions

> had historically been an *ad hoc*, reactive process, and the result was confusion, complexity, and lack of coordination. The resultant chaos was unacceptable under public funding, and the committees and commissions were an attempt to determine a rational approach to this rapidly expanding sector, to instill some order, and to establish political and administrative control before the proliferation of self-governing professions made the system totally unmanageable. (1994, 87)

The development of the regulation of the health professions will be discussed in more detail in section 2.5.

Many themes of the 1972 report – integration, moving health care out of hospitals, health promotion, and community engagement – were echoed in the *Report of the Nova Scotia Royal Commission on Health Care ("Towards a New Strategy")*, which was commissioned in 1987 and published in 1989. But there were notable differences as well. The 1989 report (Gallant) was discernibly influenced by principles of New Public Management and emphasized regionalization and decentralization, evaluatory frameworks, community engagement, and financial incentives. But it was also distinct in the approach it took to physicians. Previous reports on Nova Scotia's health care system had been written by physicians or by committees chaired by physicians. The authorship of the 1972 report included seven physicians (one of whom was the chair); the 1989 commission included one physician and was chaired by a chartered accountant. The latter report, unsurprisingly, was the first substantially to challenge the role and organization of physicians in the province. The report pointed out that in 1976 Nova Scotia had finally reached parity with the Canadian average on physician expenditure per person and that the province continued to exceed the Canadian average by ever-increasing amounts thereafter (Nova Scotia, 1989, 21). The average income for Nova Scotia physicians was by 1986 second only to Ontario physicians (20). There were, it added, simply "too many physicians in Nova Scotia" (22). "Given the trends noted above," it concluded, "there is a need to control the factors of supply, utilization, remuneration, and distribution of physicians and their services" (22).These included widening nurses' (and other health care professionals') scopes of practice; limiting the fee-for-service payment system; and restricting the issuance of new billing numbers.

It is arguable that the strategy of regionalization and decentralization undertaken by the province in the 1990s can be understood not only as part of a much larger current of thinking regarding the way in which governments ought to run public programs, but also as an attempt to wrest power away from a medical elite that was possibly one of the strongest (vis-à-vis its provincial government) in the country (Black & Fierlbeck, 2006). Nonetheless, Nova Scotia's program for health care reform was quite consistent with those being undertaken by British Columbia, Saskatchewan, Manitoba, Quebec, and New Brunswick. As Hurley et al. observe, all these health care reform commissions spoke "with one voice in arguing that current fiscal realities require a restructuring of governance to ensure better management of health care resources so that they are allocated in such a way as to obtain the most value (i.e., health) for resources expended" (1994, 494). The rationales for this move can, they add, be summarized by six themes:

> Better management will not only *contain costs*, but will produce and deliver services with *improved efficiency* in ways more *flexible and responsive* to community needs. It will improve *integration and coordination* of complementary and substitutive services, ensuring a full continuum of care available whenever possible, in a community setting and evaluated according to *health outcomes*. Finally, there is to be a significant increase in community participation in planning decisions for health care. (494)

The recommendations of Nova Scotia's 1989 report were not, however, implemented by the Conservative Buchanan government. While the incoming Conservative Cameron administration did accept most the recommendations of the report in principle, they negated any attempt at significant decentralization by proposing the establishment of six purely advisory regional health agencies appointed by the provincial government. The province did act on the report's recommendation to create a provincial health council. This body, established in 1991, was to consult with Nova Scotians and to provide the provincial government with advice on health goals and comprehensive health policy formulation. By 1992, the provincial health council had released its own report "challenging the government to act on its key recommendations" (Bickerton, 1999, 170). The Liberal opposition quickly coopted key ideas of the council's document even as the Conservative government dismissed them. On 25 May 1993, a majority Liberal government was elected, and for the first time, the province had a government with a physician as both premier (John Savage) and minister of health (Ron Stewart).

Attempts to achieve substantive reform of Nova Scotia's health care system following the establishment of public insurance can be grouped into three periods: 1994–6, 1999–2001, and 2013–15. Unsurprisingly, they follow the election of new governments: the Liberal Savage government, elected in 1993; the Conservative Hamm government, elected in 1999; and the Liberal McNeil government, elected in 2013. Interestingly, the first-ever NDP government, elected in 2009, did not propose radical structural reforms to the health care system. Rather, the Dexter government made a conscious decision not to make any profound administrative reforms on the grounds that improvements to health service delivery could be better achieved in a stable environment that was not consumed by drastic institutional restructuring (Steele, 2014b).

The first cycle of reform began directly after the inauguration of the Savage government. Health Minister Ron Stewart appointed a minister's task force (the "Blueprint Committee") which reported in the spring of 1994. The report was responding to claims that "the current focus on centralized control serves to make the system rigid, inflexible and unresponsive to regional health needs" (Nova Scotia, 1994, 6). The proposal presented by the Blueprint Committee was radical and far-ranging, but it supported the direction already articulated by both the 1989 Gallant report and the 1992 Provincial Health Council. The thrust of the Blueprint Committee's plan was the elimination of all local hospital boards and the establishment 34 community health boards (CHBs). These boards would have broad authority for the delivery of health services and the budgetary authority necessary to make extensive planning decisions. In keeping with the New Public Management dictum of "steering, not rowing," the role of the Department of Health was to be that of "planner, funder, and evaluator" making comprehensive and long-term planning decisions rather than of health provider (Nova Scotia, 1994, 10). Rather ironically, the four proposed regional health boards (RHBs) were originally designed to play a very minor role as a "communication mechanism between these two levels" (ibid, 7). In the end, however, the RHBs became the dominant players, eclipsing the CHBs altogether. As Bickerton explains, the interim regional health boards created under the framework legislation were able successfully to argue that "forcing the regional boards to share their control over regional health expenditures with community boards would be inviting disaster from a budgeting and cost-control perspective" (Bickerton, 1999, 173). Indeed, the fiscal environment in the mid-1990s was hardly a propitious time for ambitious change. By the time Ottawa introduced the 1996 Canada Health and Social Transfer, provincial health reform had completely stalled. The RHBs, comprising only members appointed by the government (and vetted by the party in power: see MacLeod, 2006, 562) were firmly in control of health service delivery. The role of the CHBs was ambivalent at best, and invisible at worst. As in other provinces, a wave of cost-cutting measures comprised health care "restructuring"; but the participatory and community-oriented thrust of the 1989, 1992, and 1994 documents was lost.

The next reform cycle was rooted in widespread public unhappiness with the cutbacks in health care services that had occurred under the label of "reform." The election of July 1999 returned a new Conservative government led by another medical doctor, John Hamm. The party had campaigned on a platform of making health care "more responsive to the community," and once elected, it immediately struck the Minister's Task Force on Regionalized Health Care in Nova Scotia (the Goldbloom report). In its public consultation phase, the task force was inundated with public criticism of the regionalization process. Nova Scotians were quite cognizant that the nature of health service delivery had changed a great deal and to no one's satisfaction; but it was unclear to the public whether the quality of health care had changed due to the structural changes or to the fiscal squeeze itself. The Goldbloom report (Nova Scotia, 1999) concluded that the structure of regionalization was essentially sound (a view supported by the province's auditor general [Nova Scotia Office of the Auditor General, 1999]), but that the roles of the RHBs and the CHBs ought to be clarified and codified in legislation. Politically, however, the government had campaigned on the principle of making health care more receptive to the needs of local communities, and simply reinforcing the status quo did not provide the optics of being politically responsive to the general public. In consequence, the government created Bill 34 (taking effect on the first of January 2001 as the Health Authorities Act), a statute that expanded the four RHBs into nine district health authorities (DHAs). It also recognized the formal existence of CHBs, although the CHBs remained purely advisory. DHAs continued to be made up of appointed members.

Despite claims by the proponents of regionalization that it would result in significant cost containment, these savings never materialized (Black & Fierlbeck, 2006). Escalating costs led the Nova Scotia government to commission a report from a private consultancy firm, Corpus Sanchez, which presented a technical discussion of the restructuring of service delivery in the province (Nova Scotia, 2007a).The suggestions – an emphasis on primary care and a move away from hospital-based care – were not particularly novel (they had, for example, already been clearly articulated in the 1972 health reform document *A New Direction for the Seventies*). Again, however, these suggestions did not translate well politically, and critics challenged the rhetoric of "change and transformation": "by change they mean reductions in the hours of service at rural ERs. By transformation they mean redefining hospitals as regional sites or community centres so they can make the argument that such sites do not need laboratory, diagnostic, surgical or even ER services" (Buott, 2008).

During the 2009 election campaign the New Democratic Party was able successfully to capitalize on the widespread public fear of the Corpus Sanchez recommendations, and it was elected on a promise not to close down rural hospitals. This was good politics but bad policy, as the rural hospital system was (as in most provinces) highly inefficient and very expensive. The political imperative to protect an economically unfeasible policy option led the government to develop an innovative solution – collaborative emergency centres (CECs) – that received much attention from jurisdictions across Canada (see chapter 4.1). But the NDP's term in office coincided with the global recession that began in 2008, and it was beset with difficult economic policy choices that, by 2013, led to the election of the McNeil Liberal government, which reamalgamated the nine DHAs into a single authority in April 2015. (See Box 2.1 for a comprehensive listing of major milestones in the development of Nova Scotia's health care system.)

Box 2.1 Major milestones in the evolution of Nova Scotia's health care system

1947   Ottawa provides a Federal Health Survey Grant to Nova Scotia to produce an inventory of the capacity of the provincial health care system.

1948   Maritime Medical Care is established.

1950   The *Report on the Survey of Hospitals in Nova Scotia under the Federal Health Survey Grant* is published.

1957   The Nova Scotia Hospital Services Planning Commission is appointed under the authority of Bill 55.

1959   Nova Scotia adopts public hospital insurance under the Nova Scotia Hospitals Act.

1966   The Advisory Commission on Medical Care Insurance is appointed under the authority of Bill 148.

1969   Nova Scotia adopts public medical insurance under the Medical Care Insurance Act.

1970   The Nova Scotia Council of Health is created (formally repealed by the Health Authorities Act in 2014).

1972   Provincial task force publishes *Health Care in Nova Scotia: A New Direction for the Seventies.*

1974   Report of the Nova Scotia Commission on Health Professional Licensing.

1989   Report of the Royal Commission on Health Care (the Gallant report).

1989   Medical Care Insurance Act and Hospital Insurance Act consolidated as the Health Services Insurance Act.

1992   Provincial Health Council releases its *Blueprint for Health.*

1994   The Minister's Action Committee on Health System Reform publishes *Nova Scotia's Blueprint for Health System Reform.*

1994   Nova Scotia passes framework legislation (the Regional Health Boards Act) to create four regional health boards.

1995   The Department of Health releases *From Blueprint to Building: Renovating Nova Scotia's Health System.*

1995   Amalgamation of four major Halifax hospitals into the Queen Elizabeth II Health Sciences Centre.

1996   The Grace Maternity Hospital and IWK Children's Hospital merge (as of 2001 the hospital becomes known as the IWK Health Centre).

1998   Emergency Medical Care (EMC), a subsidiary of Maritime
       Medical Care, is established to provide Nova Scotia's ambulance
       services.

1999   Maritime Medical Care and Blue Cross of Atlantic Canada merge
       to form Atlantic Blue Cross Care.

1999   The minister's task force publishes its report on regionalized
       health care in Nova Scotia (the Goldbloom report).

2001   The province passes the Health Authorities Act, which transforms
       the four regional health boards into nine district health authorities.

2002   The Office of Health Promotion is established.

2003   Atlantic Blue Cross Care becomes known as Medavie Inc.

2006   Province releases *Renewal of Public Health in Nova Scotia: Building a
       Public Health System to Meet the Needs of Nova Scotians.*

2006   Public health branch of the Department of Health and Chief Med-
       ical Office of Health merge with the Office of Health Promotion
       to become the Department of Health Promotion and Protection.

2007   Province releases *Changing Nova Scotia's Healthcare System: Creating
       Sustainability through Transformation* (the Corpus Sanchez report).

2010   Province releases *The Patient Journey through Emergency Care in Nova
       Scotia: A Prescription for New Medicine* (the Ross report).

2010   Province releases *Better Care Sooner: The Plan to Improve Emergency
       Care.*

2011   Department of Health merges with the Department of Health
       Promotion and Protection to become the Department of Health
       and Wellness.

2012   Nova Scotia passes the Regulated Health Professions Network
       Act.

2014   The Department of Health releases *Putting Patients First.*

2014   Nova Scotia passes the Essential Home-support Services Act.

2014   Nova Scotia passes the Essential Health and Community Services
       Act.

2014   Nova Scotia passes the Health Authorities Act.

2015   The Health Authorities Act 2014 comes into effect April 2015.
       The act amalgamates nine district health authorities into one
       (IWK remains separate).

2015   Nova Scotia passes the Public Services Sustainability Act.

2016   The Department of Health and Wellness is reorganized to reflect
       the consolidation of the DHAs.

2.2 Organization of the provincial health system

The organization of health care in Nova Scotia is formally set out in the Health Authorities Act (the Health Authorities Act 2001 was superseded by the Health Authorities Act 2014 as of 1 April 2015). In 2015 and 2016, Nova Scotia executed two major structural changes in the way that health care administration was organized. The first was an amalgamation of its nine DHAs into one large health authority (with the large women's and children's hospital in Halifax constituting a separate corporate authority). The second was an internal reorganization of the DHW, made to reflect the reamalgamation of the DHAs (see chapter 7 for a more detailed discussion of the process of reorganization).

2.2.1 The Nova Scotia Health Authority

Excepting the IWK Health Centre, the operation of Nova Scotia's health system is now under the purview of the Nova Scotia Health Authority (NSHA), which is governed by the NSHA board of directors. The IWK Health Centre for women and children in Halifax is considered a separate corporate entity. The boards of the NSHA and IWK are responsible to the DHW. The NSHA board has direct oversight of the president and CEO of the NSHA, as well as of the community health boards (see Figure 2.1). Directors on the NSHA board are now appointed directly by the minister of health and wellness, although directors on the IWK Health Centre board are self-perpetuating. The CEO of the NSHA, in turn, is responsible for eight-and-a-half vice-presidents (one VP position is shared with the IWK). The CEO and vice-presidents, in general terms, are responsible for strategic planning; quality-improvement planning; the monitoring, evaluation, and enhancement of professional service, teaching, and research; business and budget planning; developing health and wellness "integration networks" at the provincial level; and priority setting for the province.

The NSHA is further divided into four regional zones: western, northern, eastern, and central (see Figure 2.2). Each zone has both a medical executive director and an operations executive director. In general terms, all zonal executive directors are responsible for the integration and coordination of care and service within and across health care zones, ensuring compliance with provincial policy and procedure; supervising sites and service areas within their respective zones; operating within the approved service plan and budget for each respective zone;

Figure 2.1 Organizational chart of the Nova Scotia Health Authority and IWK
Health Centre, 2016

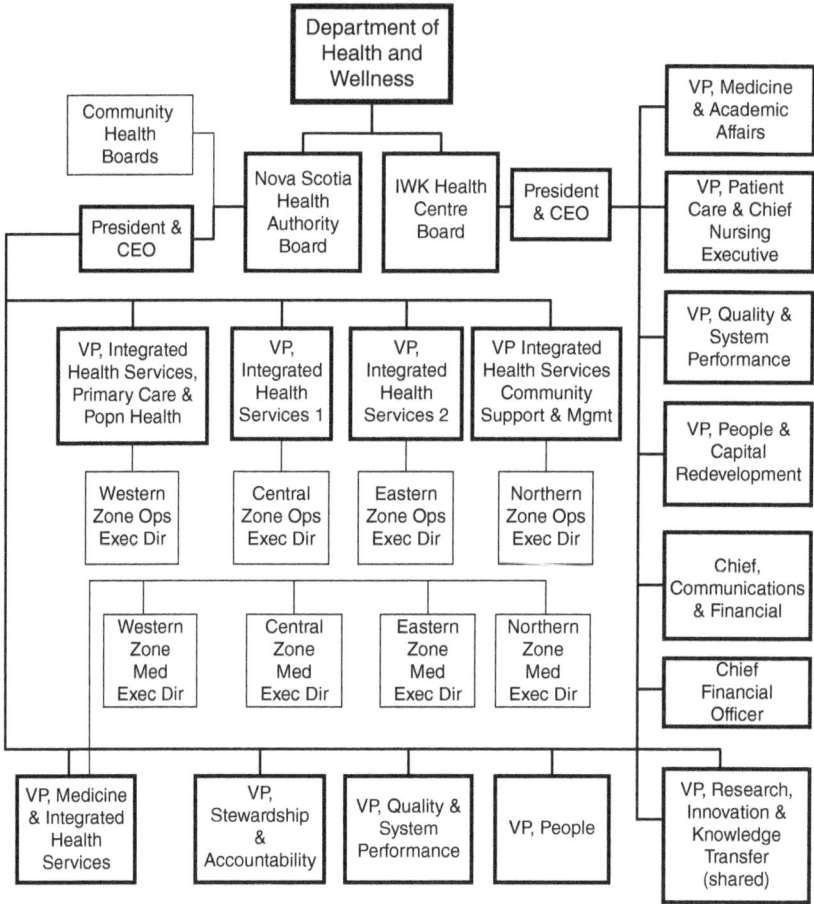

and maintaining relationships with community stakeholders. The zone medical executive directors' functions are, more specifically, to ensure consistency with provincial standards across programs and services; to develop, implement, monitor, and evaluate integrated service plans; to establish interprofessional teams; and to support the zone operations executive director. The zone operations executive directors oversee the transition and alignment of services and programs to ensure correspondence across zones; establish integrated networks within their

Figure 2.2 Nova Scotia Health Authority management zones

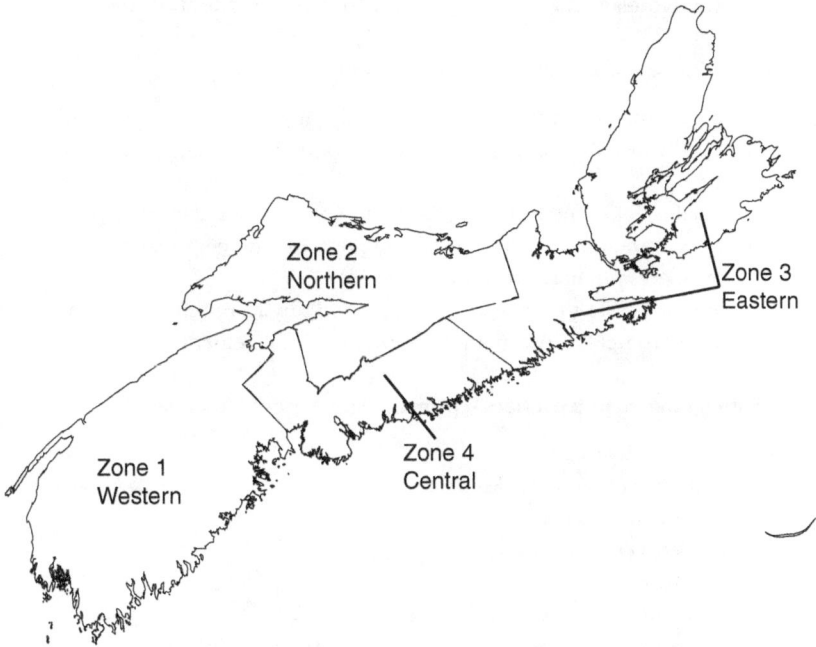

Adapted from Statistics Canada, Nova Scotia Health Regions, 2007. This does not constitute an endorsement by Statistics Canada of this product.

respective management zones; identify planning priorities; and nurture relationships with the community health boards, foundations, and auxiliary units within their jurisdictions.

The vice-presidential positions serve as the coordinating mechanism between the NSHA management and the zonal management, as well as between the NSHA and the IWK Health Centre. The VP medicine and integrated health services, for example, is a key position, as this VP directly supervises all four zonal medical executive directors and oversees physician evaluation, credentialing, remuneration, and resource planning. Each of four VPs of integrated health services has direct responsibility for the operations of one of the management zones (western, northern, eastern, and central), as well as accountability for a specific set of programs (see Box 2.2). Three VPs (stewardship and accountability, quality and system performance, and people) have no direct oversight

Box 2.2 Roles and functions of NSHA vice-presidential positions

VP medicine and integrated health services

- Provides supervision to zonal medical executive directors
- Leads the development and implementation of physician performance evaluation
- Leads development and implementation of procedural credentialing
- Oversees credentialing and privileging process and compliance
- Coordinates physician resource planning
- Represents NSHA on matters pertaining to physician remuneration
- Champions health information innovation management

VP integrated health services – primary care & population health

- Accountability for:
  - Public health and health promotion
  - Primary health care
  - Diabetes education
  - Palliative care
  - Indigenous health/first nations
  - Obstetrics and gynecology (link to IWK Health Centre)
  - Pediatrics (link to IWK Health Centre)
  - Clinical nutrition
  - Community health board support
  - Diversity
- Oversight for western zone operations

VP integrated health services – program of care 1

- Accountability for:
  - Critical care
  - Emergency/trauma
  - Laboratory medicine
  - Diagnostic imaging, pharmacy
  - Electro-diagnostics
  - Endoscopy
  - Ambulatory care clinics
  - Renal care and dialysis
- Oversight for central zone operations

VP integrated health services – program of care 2

- Accountability for:
  - Cancer care
  - Peri-operative and surgical services
  - Cardiovascular health
  - Medicine services (GI, respiratory, etc.)
  - Central sterilization and reprocessing
- Oversight for eastern zone operations

VP integrated health services – community support and management

- Accountability for:
  - Continuing care
  - Long-term care
  - Home Care
  - Seniors' care
  - Rehabilitative and psycho-social services
  - Mental health and addictions
  - Spiritual care
- Oversight for northern zone operations

VP stewardship and accountability

- Leads development and implementation of operational and business plans
- In conjunction with VP medicine, provides oversight of development and implementation of IT/IM multiyear plan
- Oversees maintenance and development of building infrastructure and asset management programs and services across the province
- Accountability for:
  - Financial transactions/operations
  - Budgeting and financial accountability
  - Information technology and infrastructure
  - Building and facility services (physical plant, maintenance, environmental services, security, grounds)
  - Procurement and logistics
  - Laundry
  - Patient food/cafeteria

- Patient transport and porter services
- Health information services
- Biomedical engineering

VP quality and system performance

- Oversees quality improvement, patient safety, risk management and system-performance systems and processes
- Accountability for:
  - Quality improvement
  - Patient safety
  - Strategic planning
  - System performance and accountability
  - Decision support
  - Policy management
  - Privacy
  - Project management
  - Infection prevention and control
  - Legal services
  - Enterprise risk management
  - Emergency preparedness
  - Accreditation planning

VP people

- Leads the design and development of a multiyear human-resources/talent-management plan
- Liaises with government, leads labour-relations strategy and implementation
- Oversees the implementation of the human resources centres of excellence resulting from shared services redesign
- Oversees organizational wellness and safety, volunteer services
- Accountability for:
  - Human resources: compensation and benefits; recruitment and staffing; talent management; employee and labour relations; employee health, safety, and wellness; HR strategy; HR operations
  - Change management
  - Public engagement, marketing and communications
  - Volunteer services

- Learner placements
- Professional practice
- Staffing/scheduling
- Employee engagement
- Organizational development

VP learning, research, and innovation (shared)

- Advises on all matters pertaining to research, innovation, and learning for both the NSHA and the IWK Health Centre
- Leads the development of a multiyear research and innovation plan with partners at the universities, community colleges, and private sector (where appropriate)
- Provides strategic and operational leadership through the development of collaborative practice environments that enable life-long learning
- Accountability for:
  - Simulation-based learning
  - Research and innovation
  - Academic health network and relationship management
  - Health, organizational and research ethics for the NSHA and the IWK Health Centre

Source: Nova Scotia Department of Health and Wellness, 2016.

role of the zones, and they focus on such matters as implementation of IT programs, infrastructure, patient safety, labour relations, and human resources.

As of 2016, the NSHA comprised a total of 45 hospitals: one tertiary (952 beds), nine regional (1,174 beds), and 35 community (1,072 beds). It had more than 23,400 employees, including 2,486 physicians and 500 residents. Its budget for 2015–16 was $1,817,546,047, which made it the largest publicly funded operation in the province (Nova Scotia Health Authority, 2015a). To assist in planning, the NSHA is supported by 37 CHBs made up of community volunteers. The 2001 Health Authorities Act gave the CHBs formal legal status, and this authority is continued under the 2014 Health Authorities Act. The purpose of CHBs under this act is to "advise the provincial health authority on local perspectives,

trends, issues and priorities, and to contribute to health-system accountability by facilitating an exchange of information and feedback between
the community and the provincial health authority." While they have
legal status, CHBs are considered to be neither corporate bodies nor
"legal entities" (and cannot therefore hire staff, hold funds indepen-
dently, or enter into contracts). The NSHA has the authority to select
members of CHBs as it sees fit, as long as the selection process is "open,
public, and transparent."

2.2.2 Contractors (private not-for-profit)

The private sector also plays a role in the administration and provision of health care in Nova Scotia. The two largest private not-for-profit
agencies playing a role in Nova Scotia's health care system are Medavie
Blue Cross (also known as Medavie Inc.), and the Health Association
of Nova Scotia (HANS). The province's relationship with Medavie is
a close and historical one. Medavie began as the Maritime Hospital
Service Association (MHSA) in 1943, offering private health insurance plans. When Nova Scotia developed its public health insurance
plan, the MHSA was asked by the province if it would be interested
in administering the new plan, but the MHSA turned down the offer,
and Maritime Medical Care was selected in its stead. The MHSA (after
changing its name to Blue Cross of Atlantic Canada in 1986) merged
with Maritime Medical Care in 1999, and was renamed Medavie Inc. in
2003. Medavie has both a "public" and a "private" persona. It offers private insurance (health, dental, vision, travel, income replacement, and
life insurance), but it also administers Nova Scotia's Medical Services
Insurance (MSI) and Pharmacare programs, as well as the health card
registration services. Because the Canada Health Act requires provincial health insurance plans to be publicly administered, the MSI plan
is formally administered and operated by a discrete body made up of
both the DHW and Medavie under section 8 of the Health Services and
Insurance Act. The current service level agreement between the DHW
and Medavie was established (without a tendered process) in 2005, with
an initial five-year contract and a number of renewal options to follow.
The contract began at $10.4 million per year, but allowed for annual
operational increases, and is in effect until March 2017 (Nova Scotia
Department of Health, 2005).

Despite Medavie's status as a not-for-profit company, it nonetheless
acts as the parent company for several for-profit companies, including

Medavie Health Services (formerly Medavie EMS Inc.), the ambulance company that was selected to provide province-wide ambulance services in Nova Scotia, and Medavie HealthEd, a private educational company that trains the paramedics that staff the ambulance services. It is not uncommon for executives to move between Medavie (the private not-for-profit body), Medavie Health Services (the private for-profit company), and public health care positions. In 2014, for example, the former president and CEO of Medavie Inc. was appointed chief administrator for the province's nine DHAs; in 2015, a former chair of the boards of both Medavie and Medavie EMS Inc. was asked to serve as the new chair of the amalgamated NSHA (after also having served as chair of the IWK Health Centre). Bernard Lord, former premier of New Brunswick, was appointed CEO of Medavie in September 2016.

Another key private not-for-profit body is HANS. This body (formerly the Nova Scotia Association of Health Authorities) performs a number of discrete functions. It interfaces with health care unions on behalf of the NSHA and the IWK Health Centre (including the negotiation of new collective agreements), and it also negotiates with health care workers on behalf of private long-term care facilities and home-care service providers. It provides medical and dental insurance to those employed by organizations it represents (such as the NSHA and the IWK) and, through the Nova Scotia Health Employees' Pension Plan (NSHEPP), it provides pensions as well. HANS also offers biomedical engineering services, including assistance regarding the acquisition of medical equipment, the coordination of clinical trials, and the inspection, repair, and disposal of medical equipment. HANS manages both the province's training program for continuing care assistants (CCAs) and a training course for those providing care to dementia patients.

In 2011, the province contracted with HealthPRO, Canada's largest health care procurement-services company, to improve the province's purchasing power in such areas as pharmaceuticals, clinical services, and food services. While the DHAs and the IWK had initially used two discrete group-purchasing organizations, they combined their purchasing under the HealthPRO contract, which continued after the amalgamation of the DHAs. Another private not-for-profit organization, Green Shield Canada, has been administering Nova Scotia's publicly insured dental programs since 2016. A number of advocacy and charitable organizations in the province also provide a wide range of health-related services (see Box 2.3).

Box 2.3 Main advocacy organizations and charities in Nova Scotia

- Active Living Coalition for Older Adults (ALCOA)
- AIDS Coalition of NS
- Alcoholics Anonymous (NS office)
- ALS Society of NB-NS
- Alternative Programs for Youth and Families
- Alzheimer Society of NS
- Autism NS
- Brain Injury Association of NS
- Brigadoon Children's Camp Society
- Cancer Care NS
- Canadian Mental Health Association (NS division)
- Canadian National Institute for the Blind (CNIB), (NS office)
- Canadian Red Cross (NS office)
- Canadian Diabetes Association (NS office)
- Canadian Paraplegic Association (NS)
- Caregivers NS
- Chebucto Community Health Team
- Child Care Advocacy Association of NS
- Community Action on Homelessness
- Continuing Care Association of NS
- Canadian Union of Public Employees (CUPE)
- Doctors NS
- Easter Seals (NS Office)
- Excalibur ADHD Association
- Family Service Association
- Feed Nova Scotia
- Heart and Stroke Foundation NS
- Hepatitis Outreach Society of NS (HepNS)
- The Huntington Society (Halifax/Dartmouth chapter)
- Immigrant Services Association of NS (ISANS)
- Laing House
- L'Arche Atlantic region
- Lung Association of NS
- Metro United Way
- Multiple Sclerosis Society of Canada (Atlantic division)
- Narcotics Anonymous (Central Nova area)

- North End Community Health Centre
- Nova Scotia Government and General Employees Union (NSGEU)
- NS Hospice Palliative Care Association
- Nova Scotia Nurses' Association (NSNA)
- Parkinson Canada (Atlantic Office)
- People First NS
- Phoenix Centre for Youth
- PrideHealth
- Prostate Cancer Canada (Halifax/Atlantic Region)
- Schizophrenia Society of NS
- Self-Help Connection
- Street Connection
- Unifor
- Victorian Order of Nurses (VON)
- YMCA
- YWCA

2.2.3 Contractors (private for-profit)

As noted above, the most prominent private for-profit organization in Nova Scotia is Emergency Medical Care Inc. (EMC), a private company run by Medavie Emergency Health Services (EHS), which is the corporate office for the private companies operated by Medavie Blue Cross (the private not-for-profit company). Somewhat confusingly, EMC Inc. is under contract to a provincial body called Emergency Health Services (EHS), which is a division of the DHW. It is not surprising that most Nova Scotians do not realize that ambulance services are a private service. (For more on ambulance services, see section 2.4.3 and chapter 6.3).

Another private company providing health services on contract to the Nova Scotia government is McKesson Canada, which has operated the telehealth service in Nova Scotia (HealthLink 811) since 2009. The service employs 29 registered nurses and cost $6.1 million in its first year. By its third year it handled more than 130,000 calls (CBC, 2010). While there is some concern that the cost per call for this service is more than twice that allocated for a GP visit in Nova Scotia, defenders claim that it eases emergency-room crowding and the demand for GP services, especially at night or on weekends, when most GP offices are closed.

McKesson Canada is a wholly owned subsidiary of McKesson Corporation, an American multinational with the 15th highest generation of revenue in the United States (Fortune, 2009).

In 2008, Nova Scotia's largest DHA at the time, the CDHA, signed an agreement with a local private company, Scotia Surgery, to permit surgeons in the public system to perform minor orthopedic surgeries at the private facility. While complex procedures such as hip replacements are still done in hospitals, the arrangement seemed to be satisfactory enough for the successive New Democratic and Liberal administrations to continue the practice. The province pays approximately $1 million per year for about 500 surgical procedures.

Halifax also has "assessment clinics" specializing in "executive health." These private companies serve both corporate businesses directly and insurance firms covering employee health care benefits. These assessments can include yearly medical exams and independent assessments of employees requesting time off work due to physical or mental health conditions. In addition to health assessments, these businesses provide injury assessment and treatment, case management, diagnostic tests, and wellness counselling. As the clinics only offer noninsured services, they are not subject to provincial regulations.

As of 2017, there are no "opted out" physicians who are practising outside the public insurance system in Nova Scotia. While neither the DHW nor the College of Physicians and Surgeons, nor Doctors Nova Scotia tracks this information, MSI (the body administering public health insurance) requires that any physicians choosing to "opt out" must inform MSI of this decision in writing. Physicians are considered to be "opted in" automatically until they actively chose to opt out, even if they are recent graduates who have never practised. MSI has not at date of writing received any such requests.

2.3 Health system planning

The Department of Health and Wellness (DHW) was formally restructured as of 1 April 2016 to reflect the 2015 amalgamation of nine DHAs into a single provincial health authority. Until the amalgamation, many services and programs (such as mental health, addictions, and cancer care) had a bifurcated nature, as there were components of these programs at both the departmental and DHA level. As a rule, the DHAs provided the services, while the DHW monitored and evaluated programs, and set standards and policy direction in these areas. The DHW also coordinated activity across DHAs as well as between the DHW, other provincial departments, community organizations, and NGOs. As of the DHW reorganization in April 2016, a considerable number of functions were transferred from the province to the Nova Scotia Health Authority. These included acute and tertiary care, mental health and addiction, primary health care, public health, and health system quality. Continuing care and clinical application management (IT) remain at the provincial level. Similarly, six programs formerly under provincial jurisdiction (Cancer Care NS, Diabetes Care Program of NS, Cardiovascular Health NS, the NS Organ and Tissue Donation Program, the NS Blood Coordinating Program, and the NS Renal Program) were transferred to the NSHA, while the Reproductive Care Program of NS and the NS Breast Screening Program were transferred to the IWK Health Centre. Only the Provincial Trauma Program and the Hearing and Speech Program remain under the aegis of the provincial government. Given that responsibility for numerous functions and programs has been shifted away from DHW, the stated function of the department is now to focus on setting strategic policy directions, priorities, and standards; measuring and monitoring health system performance; and maintaining accountability for funding. The organizational structure of the DHW is based on four discrete divisions: investment and decision support; system strategy and performance; corporate service and asset management; and client service and contract administration (Figure 2.3). As of November 2015, the chief financial officer (CFO) of the DHW, like all provincial CFOs, reports to the Department of Finance and the Treasury Board.

2.4 Coverage and benefits

Like other provinces, Nova Scotia offers public health insurance for both hospital and physician services. The Hospital Insurance Program is administered directly by the DHW, but the Medical Services Insurance (MSI) programs are administered by Medavie Blue Cross, a private not-for-profit entity, on behalf of the government of Nova Scotia (see 2.2.2). Both health insurance programs are paid through general tax revenues. No health premiums are levied directly on Nova Scotians. As in all provinces, Nova Scotia has struggled to cover more health care benefits for more groups as the federal government discontinued many forms of health care coverage for the RCMP, families of armed forces personnel, veterans, and First Nations. Health care for refugees, briefly

Figure 2.3 Internal organizational chart of the Department of Health and Wellness, 2016

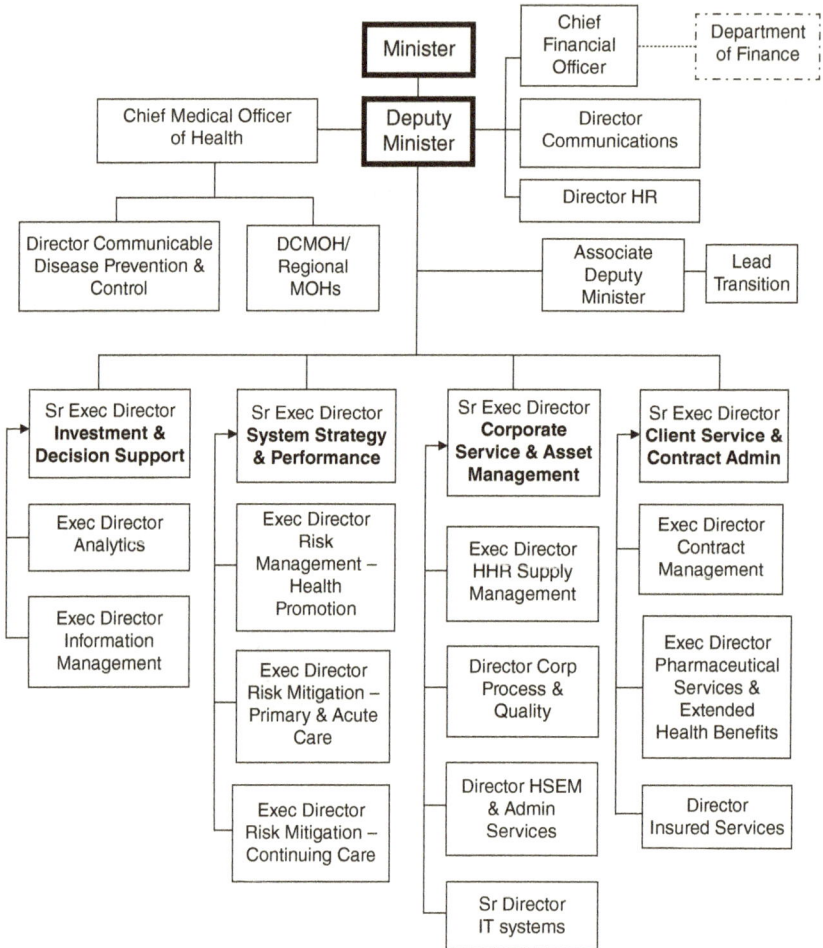

discontinued by the federal Harper administration, is again reimbursed by Ottawa.

2.4.1 Eligibility for publicly insured benefits

All Canadian citizens, or permanent residents with a permanent and principal home in Nova Scotia, are generally eligible for public health insurance, as long as they are present in the province for at least 5 months (the residency requirement until 2014 was six months, but this changed to provide more flexibility to individuals who spend the winter months outside the country). Those who are covered by federal health insurance are not eligible for provincial coverage. This category includes members of the Armed Forces (although their spouses and dependents may claim provincial health insurance) and inmates of federal penitentiaries. Canadian full-time students from other provinces are also not covered by Nova Scotia medical insurance, as they retain coverage in their home provinces. If students from outside the province have a student permit, they may apply for coverage after they have resided in the province for a year, although they may not be absent for more than 31 consecutive days.

For Canadian citizens or permanent residents moving permanently to Nova Scotia from elsewhere within Canada, public insurance coverage begins on the first day of the third calendar month following the first day of residency in the province. However, if Canadian citizens or permanent residents move permanently to Nova Scotia from outside Canada, they may claim coverage from the first day of arrival. Foreign workers with a work permit may apply for coverage on arrival in the province, although they must remain in the province for at least a year, and cannot leave Nova Scotia for more than a month. However, once deemed a resident of the province for the purpose of medical insurance coverage, individuals intending to return to Nova Scotia permanently can apply to retain their coverage while temporarily absent for up to one year.

2.4.2 Benefits (universal)

Hospital coverage is universal for all eligible individuals and covers all medically necessary care provided in a hospital. Only standard rooms are covered publicly, although room upgrades may be covered by private insurance plans. Certain services (such as physiotherapy, dental, and optometry) may be covered publicly inside a hospital, and privately outside a hospital setting. Medical services insurance provides universal coverage to all eligible individuals as long as they are provided within a "recognized clinical setting." These services include "all diagnostic, medical, psychiatric, surgical, or therapeutic procedures, including the services of anaesthetists and assistants as per the definition of medical necessity" (Nova Scotia Medical Services Insurance, Physician's Manual, 2014, 2.2.1). In Nova Scotia, "medical necessity" is defined as "those services provided by a physician to a patient with the intent to diagnose or treat physical or mental disease or dysfunction, as well as those services generally accepted as promoting health through prevention of disease or dysfunction" (ibid., 6.0.52). However, *any* services "provided in circumstances where they were not medically necessary" are not insured, and services "explicitly deemed to be uninsured" will not be covered regardless of any individual judgment about their medical necessity (ibid., 6.0.53). Both contraceptive advice and therapeutic abortion are insured services. Influenza vaccines are covered for all MSI recipients, and may be administered by qualified health professionals such as nurses and pharmacists as well as by physicians. Out-of-country health insurance is limited but is provided universally to all MSI-eligible individuals. Unsurprisingly, the most common medical service provided to Nova Scotians is a basic office visit (which in 2015 was reimbursed at $30.81 for all individuals under 65).

2.4.3 Targeted benefits for nonmedical services

Ambulance: The standard ambulance fee is Nova Scotia is $146.55 (see Table 2.3), although fees are waived for low-income patients, and costs are offset for nursing-home residents and patients with reduced mobility. Nova Scotia does not charge ambulance fares for transferring patients between health care facilities.

Dental: Nova Scotia provides no coverage for routine dental services for adults, but until 2013 it covered children ages 9 and under through the Children's Oral Health Program. In 2013, the age bracket was expanded to 13 years of age and, in 2014, it was expanded to age 14. The program was to have expanded incrementally by 1 year of age per year to age 17 in 2017, but this expansion was placed on hold in 2015 in order to review the program (see chapter 6.8). Special dental services are also provided to those who have a cleft palate, are mentally challenged, are students at the School for the Blind, or who are undergoing cranial surgery.

Nursing benefits/home care: The DHW will subsidize accommodation costs for low-income individuals who require long-term residential care, and it pays standard health care costs for all residents. The province also offers a number of home-care and caregiver programs (for more detail see chapter 6.4).

Prescription drugs: The Seniors' Pharmacare program covers residents 65 and over if they do not have private coverage. Until January 2016 seniors with an income above $18,000 paid both an annual premium ($424) as well as a co-pay of one-third of the cost of each prescription (seniors

Table 2.3 Ambulance costs in Canada, 2015

Province	Cost	
British Columbia	$50 if treated on scene; $80 if transported to hospital	
Alberta	$250 if treated on scene; $385 if transported to hospital	
Saskatchewan	Depending on the health region, $245 or $325 + $2.30/km	
Manitoba	Depending on where you are in the province, the cost ranges from $270 + $3/km to $530	
Ontario	$45 if medically necessary; $240 if not medically necessary	
Quebec	$125 + $1.75/km	
New Brunswick	In New Brunswick those without private insurance don't pay ambulance fees	
Nova Scotia	Medically essential transportation	Inter-facility transportation
Most Nova Scotians with a valid health card	$146.55	$0.00
Non-Nova Scotians	$732.95	$0.00
Non-Canadians & new Canadians	$1,099.35	$1,067.35
People who are third party insured (This includes people in a motor vehicle accident, covered by Worker's Compensation, or the federal government.)	$732.95	$711.60
Nova Scotians who are mobility challenged	$108.95	N/A
Fee to transport nursing home and residential care facility residents to hospital and back	$54.50	$0.00
Newfoundland and Labrador	$115	
Prince Edward Island	$150	
Yukon	No out-of-pocket charges to patients	
Northwest Territories	No out-of-pocket charges to patients	
Nunavut	No out-of-pocket charges to patients	

Sources: http://www.cbc.ca/marketplace/blog/map-ambulance-fees; http://www.novascotia.ca/finance/site-finance/media/finance/budget2015/2015-2016_User_Fees_and_Government_Charges.pdf

who received the federal Guaranteed Income Supplement were exempt from these premiums). The DHW attempted to change the structure of the Seniors' Pharmacare program in January 2016 so that the exemption income level for premiums increased to $22,986, with a sliding scale for premiums above this amount based on income (with a maximum premium of $1,200). In the face of a loud public outcry, however, the DHW backed down on the sliding scale for premiums.

The Family Pharmacare Program is formally available to all Nova Scotians and requires both a co-payment and deductible, which are determined according to ability to pay and family size. Drug assistance is also available for cancer patients with an income below $15,720.

The Palliative Care Drug program provides coverage for drugs required for those in palliative care at home; while the Department of Community Services Pharmacare Benefits Program provides drug coverage to those on income assistance, "Services for Persons with Disabilities" clients, children in care, and "Low Income Pharmacare for Children" clients.

Preventive services: These services are generally age related (e.g., well-baby care, vaccinations, etc.), although they can also include tests and examinations offered to individuals who have a family history of, or symptoms of, a disease that puts them at risk for preventable target conditions.

Prostheses: Mastectomy prostheses are covered up to $150 ($300 if bilateral) every 2 years; artificial limbs (with prior approval) are covered once every 4 years; and ocular prostheses are covered for residents over 18, under 65, and for those registered with CNIB.

Vision care: Corrective lenses are not covered, but one routine eye examination every 24 months is covered for those 9 years of age and younger, or 65 years of age and older.

Services not insured by MSI include cosmetic surgery, acupuncture, electrolysis, reversal of sterilization, in vitro fertilization, provision of travel vaccines, and newborn circumcision.

PRIVATE HEALTH INSURANCE

Most private health insurance in Nova Scotia, as in other provinces, covers goods and services that are not insured by the public sector. These most frequently include prescription drugs, dental and optometry services, and travel insurance. In six provinces (Alberta, British Columbia, Manitoba, Ontario, Prince Edward Island, and Quebec), private health insurers are prohibited from covering services offered under public health insurance. In Nova Scotia, however, patients of physicians who opt out of the public insurance system could substitute private for public coverage of these services; but physicians cannot charge fees that are higher than those set under public insurance.

2.5 Regulation

The regulation of health providers in Nova Scotia was, historically, a reflection of the regulatory issues within Great Britain during the eighteenth century. Unlike the French colonies in Quebec, which had required physicians to be licensed as early as 1750, the British colonies exhibited the same weak regulatory structures as Britain itself displayed, driven in large part by the intense rivalry between physicians, surgeons, and apothecaries. Moreover, as a large proportion of the physicians practising in Nova Scotia were employed by the military rather than self-employed, the relative number of "quacks" was, in comparison to Lower Canada, not perceived to be large (Marble, 1993, 168, 170, 176). Nonetheless, the quality of medical care was uneven at best, given the lack of attention placed on the accreditation of eighteenth-century physicians. As Marble notes, between 1749 and 1799, only 14 out of 366 medical practitioners in Nova Scotia had medical degrees, but even so these degrees were (as was common at the time) usually awarded without students having the burden of attending lectures or sitting exams. Indeed, within this same time period only one physician in Nova Scotia possessed a medical degree earned by attending classes and writing exams (ibid., 176). Yet the regulatory landscape changed considerably in the nineteenth century. In 1800, only 2 out of 38 medical practitioners in Nova Scotia held a medical degree, and both of these were granted without formal examination. By Confederation, 235 out of 255 of practising physicians in the province held a degree from the United States, Britain, or Lower Canada (Marble, 2006, 11).

There was an attempt by some of those practising medicine in eighteenth-century Nova Scotia to persuade the province to establish a regulatory authority for physicians. In 1797 a bill to "Regulate the Practice of Physick and Surgery" was introduced in the House of Assembly, but did not survive past second reading. After several more failed attempts, the province finally passed its first Medical Act in 1828. There was little evidence that this act was effective, however; and the fact that it was rarely enforced was due primarily to the absence of a regulatory body that had the ability to police its members. To this end, a medical society was established in 1854 (largely by Halifax physicians, many of whom had been trained within the strict Scottish medical-school system). A revised Medical Act was passed in 1856, which required physicians to register their credentials (Marble, 2006). Further revisions in 1872 allowed for the creation of the provincial medical board, which was responsible for registering and monitoring physicians' qualifications, as well as for disciplining members of the medical profession. This was the basis for the current model administered by the College of Physicians and Surgeons of Nova Scotia. Nova Scotia was also the first province to pass legislation (in 1910) governing the regulation of the nursing profession.

2.5.1 Providers

All licensed health care providers in Nova Scotia are governed by discrete statutes, each with a corresponding set of regulations (see Table 2.4). Physicians, for example, are subject to the Medical Act (formally An Act Respecting the Practice of Medicine), as well as the Medical Practitioners' Regulations established under Section 11 of the Medical Act. This act gives the College of Physicians and Surgeons of Nova Scotia the authority to regulate the medical profession in the province. In addition to the requirements set out in the Medical Act and its corresponding regulations, the college can establish policies and guidelines pertaining to the practice of medicine. "Policies" reflect the position of the college, and doctors licensed by the college are expected "to be familiar with and to comply with College policies." "Guidelines," in contrast, are simply recommendations endorsed by the college; physicians are "encouraged to be familiar with and to follow its guidelines whenever possible and appropriate" (College of Physicians and Surgeons of Nova Scotia, 2014). For example, the college has set out a *policy* on qualifications required to perform certain cosmetic procedures in Nova Scotia, has established *guidelines* on standards of care for walk-in clinics, and has articulated both policies *and* guidelines for complementary and alternative therapies. In 2012, the College of Physicians and Surgeons, the DHW, and the DHAs decided to implement a system of specialist medical credentialing in light of British Columbia's 2011 Cochrane report. The process began to be introduced in Nova Scotia in 2015.

As in most provinces, however, the structure of individual regulatory bodies for each regulated health profession presented an obstacle to collaborative activity between the health professions. For this reason, the provincial government introduced the Regulated Health Professions Network Act in 2012. While this statute protects the regulatory authority of each regulated health profession, it also facilitates the ability of these regulated professions to work together in areas such as the investigation of patient complaints, the review of decisions on licensing and registration, and the interpretation and modification of scopes of practice. While most provinces now have some form of legislation governing interprofessional collaboration in health care, the Nova Scotia statute is quite distinct because, unlike the model employed by Ontario and British Columbia, which places a "duty of collaboration" on regulatory bodies, Nova Scotia's legislation is designed to enable rather than coerce collaborative activity between regulated health professions (Lahey, 2013; Lahey & Fierlbeck, 2016).

Table 2.4 Regulatory bodies and supporting legislation

Regulatory body	Supporting legislation
College of Dental Hygienists of NS	Dental Hygienists Act
College of Licensed Practical Nurses of NS	Licensed Practical Nurses Act
College of Occupational Therapists of NS	Occupational Therapists Act
College of Physicians and Surgeons of NS	Medical Act
College of Registered Nurses of NS	Registered Nurses Act
Denturist Licensing Board of NS	Denturists Act
Midwifery Regulatory Council of NS	Midwifery Act
NS Association of Medical Radiation Technologists	Medical Radiation Technologists Act
NS Association of Social Workers	Social Workers Act
NS Board of Examiners in Psychology	Psychologists Act
NS College of Chiropractors	Chiropractic Act
NS College of Dispensing Opticians	Dispensing Opticians Act
NS College of Medical Laboratory Technologists	Medical Laboratory Technology Act
NS College of Optometrists	Optometry Act
NS College of Pharmacists	Pharmacy Act
NS College of Physiotherapists	Physiotherapy Act
NS College of Respiratory Therapists	Respiratory Therapists Act
NS Dental Technicians Association	Dental Technicians Act
NS Dietetic Association	Dieticians Act
Provincial Dental Board of NS	Dental Act
College of Paramedics of Nova Scotia	Paramedics Act

Legislation supporting the regulation of paramedics was passed in December 2015; it is in force as of April 2017. Audiologists are not regulated in Nova Scotia. Because most audiologists in the province are employed in the public school system, they are generally represented by the Nova Scotia Teachers Union.

2.5.2 Facilities

All hospitals in Nova Scotia are governed by the Hospitals Act and the regulations made under section 17 of the Hospitals Act. Clinical standards for hospitals can be monitored in more detail by Accreditation Canada, an independent not-for-profit organization. Participation in the accreditation program is voluntary, although all teaching hospitals in Canada are required by the Royal College of Physicians and Surgeons of Canada to be accredited with Accreditation Canada. Accreditation Canada bills its program as free from government intervention, although section 9 of Nova Scotia's hospital regulations stipulates that any hospital receiving a report from the agency must forward the report to the minister of health. In June 2014, the College of Physicians and Surgeons of Nova Scotia announced that it would work with the government to develop legislation regulating private health care clinics. The minister of health and wellness was quoted as saying that work on legislation would begin in the fall of 2014 (Wong, 2014), but by 2017 no further action on this matter had been taken.

2.5.3 Prescription drugs

The regulation of prescription drugs formally falls under federal jurisdiction. However, once drugs are licensed for use in Canada, provinces have the ability to determine how these drugs are used and how much they are willing to pay for them. One area of concern for the province is the misuse and diversion of prescription opioids. Nova Scotia has had a prescription-monitoring program since 1992. This program mandated the use of triplicate prescription pads for narcotic and controlled drugs. In response to the considerable increase in the abuse of prescription opioids beginning in the late 1990s, Nova Scotia enacted the Prescription Monitoring Act in 2004. This statute established the Nova Scotia Prescription Monitoring Board with a mandate to develop and operate a web-based prescription-monitoring program. Under this legislation, prescribers, pharmacists, and law-enforcement officials can access detailed information on patients' use of monitored pharmaceuticals. The program can also provide "peer-prescriber" comparator reports so that prescribers can compare their rates of narcotic prescribing with others throughout the province. "Overprescribers" can be referred to the program's Practice Review Committee for review, and this body can forward any file to a licensing body (of physicians, pharmacists, or dentists) for further review (see chapter 6.5). The program is administered by Medavie Blue Cross.

In 2011, Nova Scotia passed the Fair Drug Pricing Act. This statute allowed Nova Scotians within the provincial pharmacare program to pay steadily decreasing rates for generic drugs. By July 2012, prices for generic drugs were capped at 35 per cent of the brand-name price. The legislation also allows the government to tender for drugs as well as limit or require the reporting of rebates paid to pharmacists by drug manufacturers, although the government has not to date used these measures.

2.5.4 Patient health information

Nova Scotia's Personal Health Information Act came into effect in 2013. This act governs the collection, utilization, and disclosure of personal health information. All health care professionals regulated by the province are subject to the act, as are any other individuals or organizations entrusted with personal health information (e.g., licensed nursing homes). The "custodians" of such information are accountable for the way in which this information is used, and must engage in safeguards that protect clients' information. Individuals have a right to access their own health information, to request a correction of this information if required, to request a record of anyone who has accessed this information, and to be notified if there has been a breach of this information *if* there is the "potential for harm or embarrassment" to the individual. The act also sets out the terms and conditions under which personal health information can be used for research purposes. Somewhat confusingly, there is also federal privacy legislation (the Personal Information Protection Electronic Documents Act), which applies to the delivery of health services considered to be commercial. As the provincial privacy law has been deemed to be "substantially similar" to the federal legislation, however, commercial health care providers are now expected to comply only with the provincial Personal Health Information Act.

2.6 Patients

The idea of a "Patients' Bill of Rights" had been considered by the Hamm government, which had asked the Provincial Health Council to develop this concept in more detail. But the council, reporting in 2000, noted that a legislated patients' rights document would be too complex and problematic. In its place, the council produced a document entitled "Expectations for Health and Health Care in Nova Scotia," which outlines what the citizens of Nova Scotia can reasonably expect of their health care system, both at a system-wide level and from the perspective of individuals accessing health care services. Both sets of expectations were written at a very high level of generalization: the first category, for example, included "the development and delivery of service that reflects a commitment to the health, general well-being and dignity of all residents" as well as "the development and delivery of service guided by the best available qualitative, quantitative, and experiential evidence"; while the second category noted that individuals interacting with the health care system could expect to be "treated with respect, dignity, and consideration" with attention being paid to their "views, preferences, observation and problems regarding all aspects of care." None of these provisions are justiciable.

Until 2015, individual DHAs also produced sets of "rights" for patients within their catchment areas. The Capital Health District Health Authority, for example, produced a list of patient rights *and* responsibilities. These rights ranged from the general ("to receive the best and safest health care possible") to the specific ("to know the names, positions, titles and professional relationships of those on your health care team," "to know and understand the risks and benefits of any medicine, treatment, or decision about your health"). Responsibilities included "following the treatment plan as agreed to with your physician or health care team" and "notifying your physician or health care team of any changes in your health." Under the 2005 Involuntary Psychiatric Treatment Act, individuals "experiencing a loss of freedom to make their own decisions" (e.g., those undergoing involuntary psychiatric assessment or subject to a declaration of involuntary admission) can access an advisor who will explain why they have lost their ability to make their own decisions, the options available to have this decision reviewed, and how they may obtain formal legal representation.

Patient complaints are generally divided into two categories: complaints related to health care professionals and complaints related to institutional or systemic issues. Complaints against health care professionals can be levied through their professional associations. Until 2015, complaints pertaining to institutional or systemic issues before the amalgamation of health districts were made through the relevant health authority. Larger DHAs tended to have formal institutionalized mechanisms for processing such complaints. The CDHA, for example, had used the Patient Experience Reporting System (PERS) since 2011. This allowed the DHA to track complaints by location, type, and severity. In the 2012–13 fiscal year, the CDHA received 1875 complaints. Most fell in the low-to-moderately severe category, and most dealt with issues of poor communication and lack of empathy (Capital District Health Authority, 2014a). Similarly, patient engagement initiatives were usually undertaken at the DHA level. The CDHA, for example, initiated a citizen engagement policy in 2010. The stated aim of the policy was to "ensure decisions and priorities reflected the needs of those served by Capital Health," to "create sustainable trust relationships between Capital Health and patients and citizens," and to "ensure Capital Health was open to diverse opinions and ideas, and transparent with its information, actions, and decisions" (Capital District Health Authority, 2014b). The projects undertaken within this initiative included citizen and patient engagement regarding food options sold in the DHA's facilities; prenatal and postpartum care; the decommissioning of facilities; fiscal priorities; and health care quality and patient safety.

Both patient complaints regarding health services and patient engagement are now addressed by the NSHA.

2.7 Summary

Until the implementation of health insurance in the 1960s, health care in Nova Scotia was a largely local matter. Once health insurance was established, the issue of cost became preeminent, and the province began to consider system-wide organizational changes. Public reports on health care published by the province in 1972, 1989, and 1999 all recommended some version of a more regionalized system, with regional health authorities integrating local services and answering to a central authority. The province established four regional health authorities in 1994; these were expanded to nine district health authorities in 2001, and collapsed into a single provincial health authority in 2015. This latest reform attempts to balance attention to local need and knowledge, on the one hand, with consistency and the efficient allocation of resources across regions, on the other hand. To this end, a zonal structure has been employed. As in most regionalized systems, the objective is to distinguish between the provision of services (currently through the NSIIA) and the development of policymaking (under the aegis of the Department of Health and Wellness). There is, however, still some lack of clarity regarding precisely where the responsibility for certain aspects of health care provision (e.g., physician services) resides (see chapter 8). These tensions will have to be resolved as the new system matures and addresses specific challenges on an ongoing basis.

Chapter Three

Health Spending and Financing

Expenditure on health care in Canada as a proportion of public spending increased steadily from the introduction of public health insurance, and by 2016 it stood at 11.1 per cent of GDP (CIHI, 2016a, 6). This, in and of itself, is not a concern; while the health care system is increasingly expensive, it also provides more (and more effective) treatments and services. Higher spending, in this way, often reflects the value that societies place on improving medical care for their citizens (Reinhardt, 2015). Moreover, while spending on health care keeps increasing, the *rate* of growth has slowed noticeably since 2010, barely keeping pace with inflation and population growth (CIHI 2016a).

Nevertheless, the fiscal sustainability of public health care remains an issue. Canada is one of the highest spenders on health care in the Organisation for Health Development (OECD) (CIHI, 2016a), and there is concern that specific cost drivers (such as pharmaceutical costs and demographic shifts) may place significant pressures on provincial governments. There is considerable debate regarding precisely how important these cost drivers are. Genome-based medical treatments have produced very expensive drugs (largely in oncology) that strain the public capacity to provide them (O'Sullivan, Orenstein, & Milla, 2013). At the same time, Canada's population is steadily aging, with those over 65 now outnumbering those under 15. Yet the consequences of these cost drivers are not definite. Pharmaceutical costs, for example, are the result of specific political and regulatory contexts that are often determined as much by political will as other variables (Morgan, Law, Daw, Abraham, & Martin, 2015). And while the trend towards an increasing number of older adults is clear, the link between age and health care expenditure is not. Health care costs in Canada do increase significantly for those over 80 (CIHI, 2016a, 22), but the reasons for this increase can reflect a number of different causes, including "provider systems, incentives, approaches to interventions in frail older people, and cultural norms, particularly near the time of death," rather than simply a biological imperative (WHO, 2015, 96). The "compression of morbidity" thesis, for example, suggests that poor health is increasingly condensed into a shorter period at the end of life (Fries, 1980; Nusselder, 2002). In this reading, high end-of-life costs are largely due to the political unwillingness to discontinue expensive but ineffective treatments given at the end of a natural lifespan. Moreover, Evans, McGrail, Morgan, Barer, and Hertzman (2001) argue that an aging population can be used as a convenient excuse for increasing health care costs, drawing attention "away from questions as to the appropriateness or effectiveness of patterns of care provision, or of the levels of income they generate."

There is thus considerable disagreement on the role of aging as a cost driver in health care expenditure. CIHI (2011, 2016a) notes that population aging in Canada is only a modest cost driver overall, accounting for only 1 per cent of cost increases annually. Other economists, however, warn that the consequences of an aging population include not only more elderly adults (the expenditure effect) but also fewer individuals in the labour force (GDP effect) and the availability of more expensive diagnostics and treatments (service intensity) (Richards & Busby, 2015). In this reading, the economic impact of aging may in fact be greater than acknowledged.

What is certain, however, is that the constraints placed on health care expenditure by an aging demographic in Canada are much more pronounced in the Atlantic provinces. In Nova Scotia, as in New Brunswick, 18.3 per cent of the population was aged 65 or older in 2014, compared to 11.4 per cent in Alberta and 15.6 per cent in Ontario (Statistics Canada, 2014). As this chapter describes, the fiscal pressures of aging for Nova Scotia's health care system are important given an economic context of stagnant growth and, as some have argued, in a political context of federal health care transfers "biased against provinces with above-average rates of population aging" (Ruggieri, 2015; see also Saillant, 2016).

3.1 Health expenditure and trends

Speaking to the Halifax Chamber of Commerce before the release of the 2015 budget, Nova Scotia Finance Minister Diana Whalen asked rhetorically, "What do you do when you run out of taxpayers?" Nova

Table 3.1 Provincial economic and health data for Nova Scotia, 2000–14

	2000	2010	2014
GDP at market prices (current $, millions)	29,962	35,693	37,659
Population	933,821	942,073	942,387
GDP per capita (current $)	32,085	35,888	39,961
Government revenues ($ thousands)	5,146,912	9,269,665	10,266,529
Government revenues per capita ($)	5,511.67	9,839.65	10,894.18
Total health spending per capita (current $)	3,037.42	6,160.04	6,760.99
Total health spending as % of GDP	11.1	15.7	15.6
Share of Nova Scotia health spending as a per cent of total of government spending including debt repayment (%)	31.5	38.1	39.9
Share of Nova Scotia health spending as a per cent of total of government spending excluding debt repayment (%)	39.1	42.0	43.8

Source: Statistics Canada, 2014 (CANSIM Tables 384–0038 and 051–0001); Nova Scotia Department of Finance, Public Accounts (2000, 2010, and 2014b); CIHI National Health Expenditure Trends, Tables B.4.1, B.1.2, and B.1.3.

Scotia's demographics, as the minister noted, placed the province in a highly untenable position, as the emigration of skilled labour to other provinces meant both a higher proportion of older adults placing more demands on the health care system and a smaller proportion of taxpayers able to support these services. Given a small and beleaguered economy constrained by structural limitations, she argued, the province is increasingly unable to provide services and programs "built for a time that no longer exists" (Withers, 2015). Some public policy analysts have expressed similar concerns (Saillant, 2016). Regardless of whether one holds that such expressions of crisis in Nova Scotia's fiscal situation are exaggerated or not, the level of health expenditure relative to revenue capacity is nonetheless sobering (Table 3.1).

For example, both Alberta and Nova Scotia spend close to the same amount per capita on health care ($6,783 and $6,761, respectively, in 2014). Expressed as a percentage of GDP, however, health expenditure in Nova Scotia (at 15.6 per cent) is almost twice as high as that in Alberta (8.0 per cent) (CIHI, 2014, Table B.1.3). As discussed in chapter 1, Nova Scotia faces an extraordinary array of cost drivers. A key variable is the proportion of the population over 65: in Nova Scotia, one in seven inhabitants is over 65; in Alberta, the ratio is one in 10. A higher proportion of those over 65, in turn, means higher rates of chronic disease, a higher utilization of primary care services, and greater consumption of

Table 3.2 Health expenditure by use of funds in Nova Scotia, 2015 and forecast 2017

Category	2015			2017 (forecast)		
	Expenditures ($ millions)	Percentage distribution	$ per capita	Expenditures ($ millions)	Percentage distribution	$ per capita
Hospitals	2103.3	33	2229.52	2161.5	32.5	2272.36
Other institutions	833.6	13.1	883.64	852.8	12.8	896.52
Physicians	820.1	12.9	869.35	840.7	12.6	883.88
Other professionals	547.5	8.6	580.37	587.9	8.8	618.05
Drugs	1051.9	16.5	1115.00	1114.0	16.7	1171.14
Capital	83.8	1.3	88.87	106.9	1.6	112.41
Public health	154.4	2.4	163.69	150.7	2.3	158.45
Administration	217.7	3.3	222.09	217.7	3.3	228.86
Other health spending	569.9	8.9	604.07	622.1	9.3	653.99
Total	6374.0	100.0	6756.60	6654.3	100.0	6995.66

Source: National Health Expenditure Database, CIHI (2017), CIHI, 2017, D series data tables.

pharmaceuticals. When home-care, long-term-care, and palliative-care systems are underdeveloped, it can also mean a higher utilization of high-cost hospital beds. A second factor explaining the high cost of health care in Nova Scotia is the distribution of population density. It is much more cost-efficient to provide health care services in population-dense urban areas. High-cost services requiring an element of specialization (such as obstetrics) are simply more expensive to provide in smaller communities for a number of reasons, including not only the logic of scale economies but also incentives to health professionals to work in smaller centres. Nova Scotia has only one "urban centre" (defined by Statistics Canada as a community of 100,000 and over): Halifax Regional Municipality. It also has only one population centre designated as "medium" sized (30,000 to 99,999 inhabitants): Cape Breton (even though the population of Cape Breton is spread out over a much larger area). The remaining 35 of Nova Scotia's 37 population centres are classified as "small" communities (1,000 to 29,999 inhabitants).

As outlined in Table 3.2, the majority of health care spending is on hospitals, followed by drugs and physicians. This is similar to the pattern of spending across all provinces and territories (five provinces spend a greater proportion of their respective GDP on drugs than on physicians; the reverse is true in the remaining jurisdictions). Compared to other provinces, the distribution of health expenditure across spending categories is remarkable in only one area: spending on pharmaceuticals.

The only provinces that spend more on drugs per capita than Nova Scotia are New Brunswick and Quebec. Even so, the relative proportion of health spending on pharmaceuticals in Nova Scotia has declined slightly. This may be due to a number of new strategies, including centralizing provincial drug procurement across health authorities (through HealthPRO), limiting the price paid for generic drugs, restricting the pricing methods used by pharmacies, and participating in the pan-Canadian Pharmaceutical Alliance. Moreover, many patents on commonly used drugs have expired since the mid-2000s, permitting the entry of lower-priced genetic drugs. Again, demographic variables are quite relevant. For example, anti-TNF (anti-inflammatory) drugs alone accounted for 54.8 per cent of the growth in public health spending in Canada between 2007 and 2012 (CIHI, 2013). Anti-TNF drugs are used primarily in the treatment of arthritis. The Arthritis Society notes that 23.4 per cent of Nova Scotians report having arthritis, compared to 17.5 per cent of Ontarians and 14.9 per cent of Albertans (Public Health Agency of Canada, 2011). The second drug that contributed most to the growth in pharmaceutical spending over this period was the class of antineovascularization agents used to treat age-related macular degeneration, a condition that normally occurs in the sixth or seventh decade of life, thus disproportionately affecting provinces with older populations (CIHI, 2013).

These trends in spending on specific health care categories also explain larger patterns in public and private expenditure in Nova Scotia. Both public and private expenditure have increased since 2011, but private expenditure has increased more slowly. As most private health care spending is used for pharmaceuticals (CIHI, 2014, 39) a slower rate of growth in pharmaceutical spending would also contribute to a slower growth in overall private health care spending. Conversely, relatively higher spending on hospitals and physicians means a slight growth in public vis-a-vis private health care spending. Overall, Nova Scotia's ratio of public to private health care spending (69.5 per cent to 30.5 per cent in 2014, respectively) closely reflects Canada's ratio of 70 per cent to 30 per cent. (See Table 3.3 for a comparison of total spending and public spending in Nova Scotia and Canada.) Interestingly, however, expressed as *per capita* health expenditure, private spending on health care in 2014 was higher in Nova Scotia (at $2,065) than in any other Canadian province (Figure 3.1). This can be at least partly explained by Figure 3.2, which shows that Nova Scotians spend considerably more on private health insurance premiums. This, in turn, is probably because provincial public plans are more limited in both scope and coverage

Table 3.3 Health expenditure in Nova Scotia and Canada, 2000–15 ($ millions, current dollars)

Year*	Nova Scotia		Canada	
	Total spending	Public spending**	Total spending	Public spending
2000	2,836.6	1,968.4	98,609.7	69,274.7
2001	3,013.3	2,082.7	107,201.2	74,984.5
2002	3,306.8	2,264.3	115,056.5	79,909.2
2003	3,595.8	2,484.1	123,591.4	86,566.1
2004	3,722.0	2,585.0	131,555.2	92,039.6
2005	4,026.8	2,819.0	140,196.5	98,266.1
2006	4,468.9	3,135.3	150,625.1	104,961.4
2007	4,764.2	3,351.0	160,142.4	112,372.4
2008	5,014.5	3,529.9	171,941.2	121,309.5
2009	5,279.7	3,617.9	181,971.4	129,033.6
2010	5,803.2	3,935.1	193,159.6	136,058.9
2011	6,009.1	4,184.7	199,228.6	140,846.7
2012	6,040.7	4,219.0	205,443.0	145,100.5
2013	5,956.0	4,211.7	209,457.6	148,143.4
2014	6,051.4	4,290.3	215,708.0	152,767.1
2015	6,197.2	4,390.4	215,708.0	155,000.3

*2014 and 2015 are forecasted values.
**Total public sector includes provincial/territorial, federal direct, and municipal
   governments; workers' compensation boards; and the Quebec Drug Insurance Fund.
Source: National Health Expenditure Database, CIHI (2015c), B series data tables.

than most other public provincial plans in Canada. Overall public per capita expenditure, as noted earlier, is higher than the Canadian average, though not the highest in Atlantic Canada (Figure 3.3).

3.2 Public revenue

The main sources of own-source revenue for Nova Scotia are individual income tax and consumption taxes (sales taxes). A substantial proportion of Nova Scotia's public revenues are derived from federal transfer payments, although that amount is shrinking. In 2000, federal transfers amounted to 37 per cent of total provincial revenues; by 2015 they had dropped to 30 per cent (Table 3.4).

Declining federal transfers are thus of particular concern to the province. In 2011 the federal government announced that it would revise the formula for allocating health transfers to the provinces. When Ottawa reduced direct cash transfers to the provinces in 1977 in favour of the transfer of tax points, the formula it used to calculate the remaining

Figure 3.1 Private sector per capita health expenditure by province and for Canada, 2000–13 (current dollars)

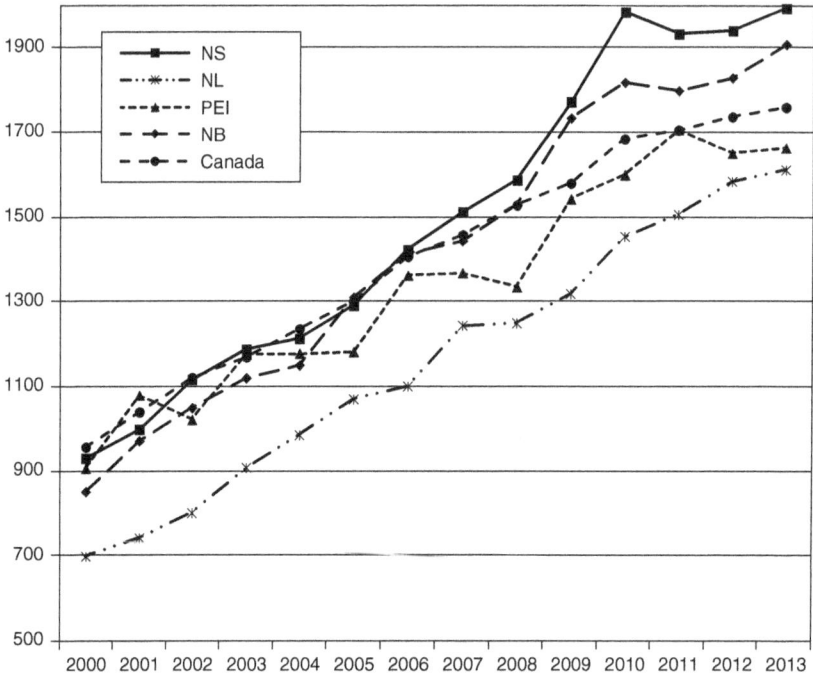

Source: National Health Expenditure Database, CIHI (2014), B series data tables.

cash portion took into account that each tax point given to wealthier provinces was worth more than one given to poorer provinces. This combination of tax-point transfers and adjusted cash transfers was intended to bring the combined value of each province's transfers to the national average. Under the revised formula announced in 2011, Ottawa now uses a strict per-capita calculation for the health transfer. This means significant reductions for Nova Scotia. In 2016–17, for example, a $947.8 million cash transfer (Canada Health Transfer [CHT]) is offset by a $23.5 million reduction in tax-point equalization. In the following year, the $1010.3 million cash transfer will see a $41 million reduction (Table 3.5). Over the period 2015–16 to 2023–24, "per capita cash increases total about $312 million, while the losses from tax point equalization are almost three times that – $775 million" (Starr, 2015). The Canadian Institute of Actuaries presents the consequences of this

Figure 3.2 Private sources of health revenue by province and for Canada, 2000–13 (current dollars)

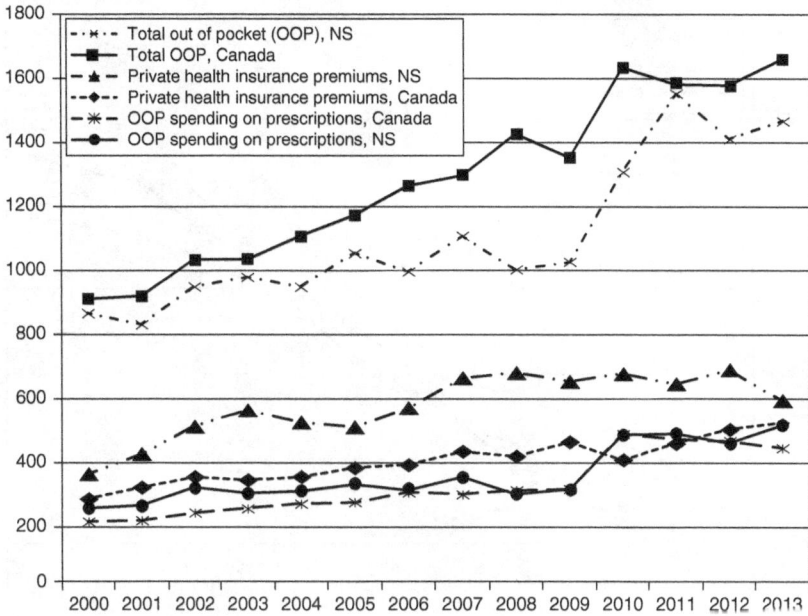

Source: Statistics Canada, Survey of Household Spending, Tables 203-0008 and 203-0021.

shift in the calculation of the CHT in a slightly different format: in 2012, health care expenditures in Nova Scotia amounted to 45.9 per cent of total revenues, or 68.5 per cent of own-source revenue. By 2020, if the rate of health care expenditure increases at current levels, health care expenditure will amount to 80.4 per cent of own-source revenues given the decline in federal transfers. Projected to 2037, health care expenditure would amount to a rather shocking 110.3 per cent of own-source revenues (Levert, 2013, 85).

In December 2016, Nova Scotia made a bilateral deal with the federal government that comprised $287.8 million over 10 years for targeted home care ($157 million) and mental health care ($130.8 million) funding.

3.3 Public financing flows

Most health care services are provided directly by the Nova Scotia Health Authority and the IWK Health Centre, which together utilize 42 per cent

Figure 3.3 Public sector per capita health expenditure by province and for Canada, 2000–13 (current dollars)

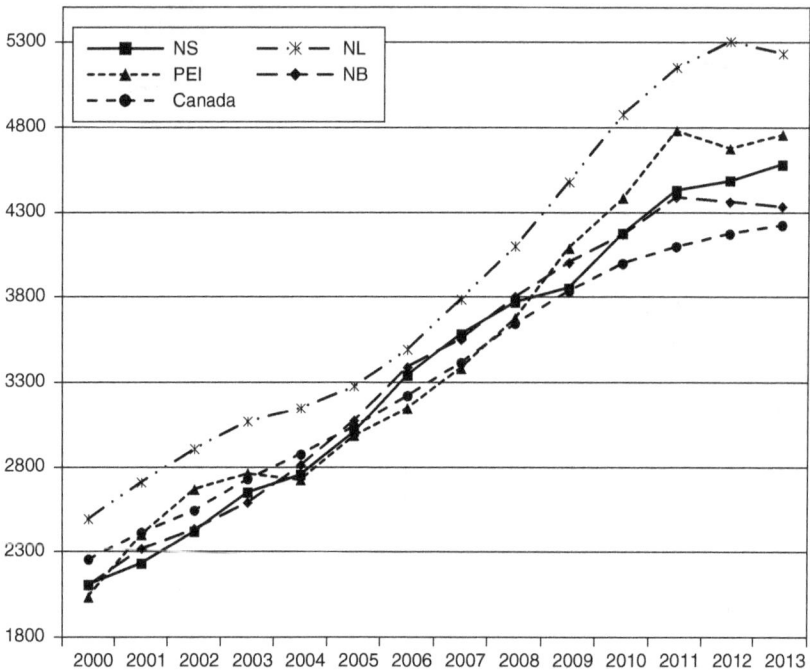

Source: National Health Expenditure Database, CIHI (2014), B series data tables.

of the health care financing provided by the provincial government. After the health authorities, the largest proportion of financing is channeled to physicians. Other programs requiring significant resources include long-term care, home care, pharmaceutical services, and emergency health services (see Figure 3.4).

Most health care expenditure by the province is quite straightforward. One notable exception is the payment methods used for physicians. As in most provinces, the payment system historically was based on a fee-for-service structure in which physicians were reimbursed for each particular medical procedure they provided. For more than a hundred years, physician reimbursement in Nova Scotia was calculated according to a fee schedule. Fee schedules in Nova Scotia prior to 1861 were largely determined by local physicians (a doctor in Halifax in 1854, for example, could appropriately charge between five shillings and one pound five shillings for a basic consultation). When the Medical Society

Table 3.4 Public sources of revenue ($ thousands)

Year	Own-source revenue		Federal transfers	
2000	Income taxes	1,294,250	Equalization payments	1,279,610
	Sales taxes	1,073,360	Equalization Offshore Revenue Offset	2,100
	Other revenue	218,310	Canada Health and Social Transfer	527,920
			Federal compensation for harmonization	52,700
			Other federal payments	41,294
	Total own-source: 2,585,920		**Total transfers: 1,903,624**	

Prior years' adjustments – federal/provincial fiscal adjustments: 9,400
Other revenue: 431,006
Sinking fund and public debt retirement fund earnings: 216,962
Total revenue: 5,146,912

Year	Own-source revenue		Federal transfers	
2010	Income taxes	2,210,469	Equalization payments	1,464,935
	Sales taxes	1,650,411	Offshore Accord	180,072
	Petroleum royalties	125,634	Wait Times Reduction Fund	6,956
	Other revenue	1,016,865	Canada Health Transfer	700,137
			Canada Social Transfer	301,978
			Other federal sources	586,163
	Total own-source: 5,003,379		**Total transfers: 3,240,241**	

Total revenue: 8,243,620

Year	Own-source revenue		Federal transfers	
2015	Income taxes	2,877,512	Equalization payments	1,750,653
	Sales taxes	2,305,426	Offshore Accord	64,481
	Petroleum royalties	33,086	Canada Health Transfer	860,397
	Other revenue	2,030,280	Canada Social Transfer	334,734
			Other federal sources	369,658
	Total own-source: 7,255,304		**Total transfers: 3,379,923**	

Total revenue: 10,635,227

Source: Finance and Treasury Board, Nova Scotia. Public Accounts, 2000, 2010, and 2015.

Table 3.5 Canada Health Transfer projections for Nova Scotia ($ millions)

	2015–16	2016–17	2017–18	2018–19	2019–20	2020–21	2021–22	2022–23	2023–24
Equal per-capita cash	902.0	947.8	979.3	1010.3	1041.3	1072.4	1102.9	1133.3	1164.0
Cash plus tax points	924.9	971.3	1020.3	1071.7	1125.7	1182.4	1241.8	1304.1	1369.6
Gap	(22.9)	(23.5)	(41.0)	(61.4)	(84.4)	(110.0)	(138.9)	(170.8)	(205.6)

Source: Broten, 2014: *Charting a Path for Growth* (the Broten Report). http://www.novascotia.ca
/finance/docs/tr/Tax_and_Regulatory_Review_Nov_2014.pdf

Figure 3.4 Nova Scotia public financing to health system, 2014–15

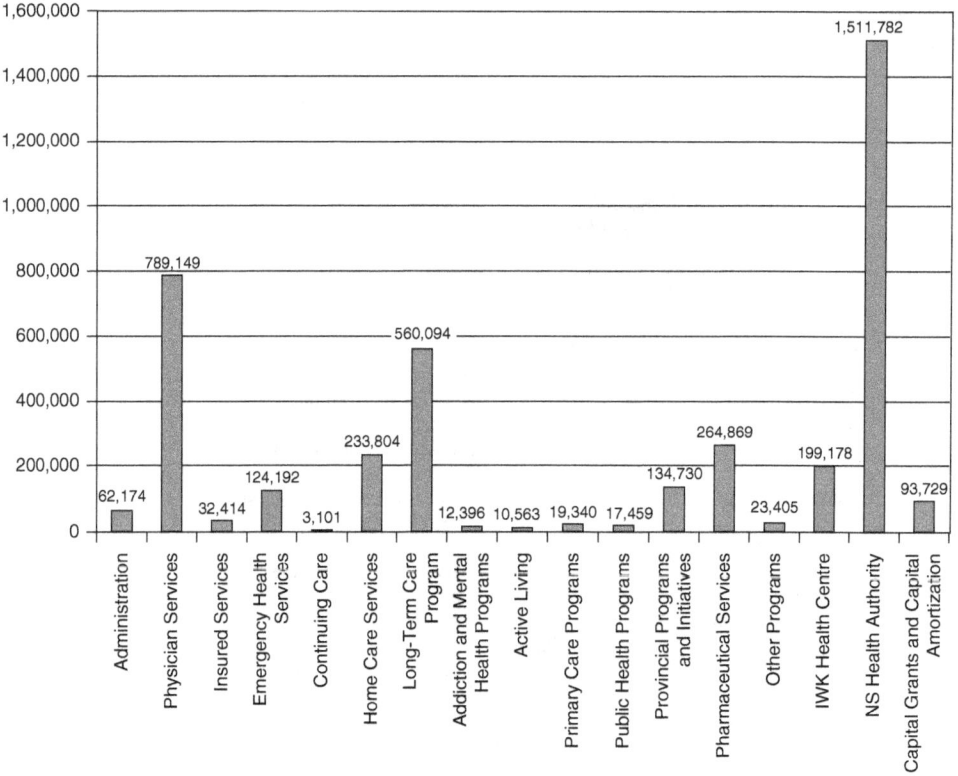

Source: Finance and Treasury Board, Nova Scotia. Budget Documents (Estimates and Supplementary Detail), 2015–2016. Available at http://www.novascotia.ca/finance/en/home /budget/budgetdocuments/default.aspx

of Nova Scotia was incorporated in 1861, it established the first province-wide fee schedule (Marble, 2006). With the advent of Medical Insurance in 1969, doctors could no longer bill patients directly for insured services. Rather, they submitted billings to the province, for which they were remunerated according to the fee schedule negotiated between the Medical Society (now Doctors Nova Scotia) and the province. However, the province does not reimburse physicians directly. Rather, Nova Scotia has contracted with Medavie Blue Cross to administer payments to physicians (and to monitor these payments). Of the 2,830 physicians currently working in Nova Scotia, approximately 51 per cent are paid on a strict fee-for-service basis (compared to the national average of 71 per cent paid fee-for-service) (CIHI, 2015b, 10).

Some physicians prefer the fee-for-service mechanism because of the flexibility and freedom it affords: each individual doctor under this system can determine, within the parameters outlined by their professional association, how they choose to practise medicine and how many hours they wish to work. But Nova Scotia has gradually been shifting away from fee-for-service payment methods to alternative payment methods. In 2014–15, out of 2,426 physicians, 703 (29 per cent) were paid 90 per cent or more through fee for service; 498 (20.5 per cent) were paid between 50 and 90 per cent through fee for service; 203 (8.4 per cent) were paid between 50 and 90 per cent through alternative payment programs; and 1,022 (42.1 per cent) were paid 90 per cent or more through alternative payment programs (CIHI, 2016b, Table A.2.3).

There are two discrete kinds of alternative payment programs in Nova Scotia. Academic Funding Plans (AFPs) had a value of approximately $213,000,000 in 2015–16, while alternative payment plans (APPs) were worth $41,000,000. During the same period, fee-for-service payments amounted to about $303,000,000 (Nova Scotia, 2016a, 13.8). AFPs were designed to enhance the recruitment and retention of specialists, and the payments cover the research, teaching, and administrative duties that academic physicians perform in addition to clinical services. The functions of APPs are quite distinct. They are used primarily to attract physicians to rural communities that have experienced difficulty in recruiting and retaining family physicians (more than 10 per cent of Nova Scotians do not have a family doctor). Pure APPs, which are standardized throughout the province, guarantee physicians in small communities a defined income regardless of the number of patients that they see; this is especially important for small communities where total billings per physician may be much smaller than in urban settings. At the same time, APP contracts specify outcomes (such as the number of hours worked or services performed) that physicians must deliver. APPs are also useful when determining contracts for collaborative work environments, where fee-for-system mechanisms are difficult to reconcile with collaborative activity. Some physicians may choose a blended system that incorporates elements of both plans; and they may choose to opt out of an APP after a three-month trial period.

But alternative payment systems are not unproblematic. They are, in the first place, quite complex to negotiate, as the contracts are negotiated between not only physicians and the Department of Health and Wellness but also with the health authority and Doctors Nova Scotia. Second, alternative payment systems are expected to perform two potentially conflicting functions: on the one hand, they are designed to attract physicians to areas where the standard rate of compensation may not be high enough to entice a doctor to settle; on the other hand, they are specifically designed to minimize the potential for overpayment that characterizes fee-for-service payment systems. Indeed, the 1997 alternative payment system clearly specified that "payments should typically draw no more resources from the Medical Services Insurance (MSI) budget/allocation than was historically drawn by fee-for-service," and yet an audit conducted in 2000 found that these alternative payment contracts were in fact costing more than the historical fee-for-service payments (Nova Scotia Office of the Auditor General, 2014b). But the biggest problem is the lack of clear performance targets and the poor monitoring of alternative payment systems. As the 2014 auditor general's report succinctly stated,

> Alternate payment plans have limited reporting requirements making it difficult for the Department to determine if an appropriate level of service is provided. When physicians paid through academic funding plans submit reports on contract deliverables, no review is completed. If the Department becomes aware that reporting requirements are not met, it does not take steps to achieve compliance ...
>
> Although progress has been made towards the development of new alternative payment and academic funding models, considerable work is still needed. (ibid., 13)

3.4 Summary

Nova Scotia faces a daunting economic situation. It has among the highest levels of health expenditure relative to revenue capacity, and financial demands on the health care system are likely to increase even as economic productivity and job-growth performance continue to stagnate (for a more detailed account of this dynamic, see Saillant, 2016). Public insurance plans are generally more restrictive than in most other provinces, and private health care spending is higher per capita even though Nova Scotians' income is lower than the national average. As general health indicators in the province are mostly poorer than those in other provinces, demands on the health care system will continue to be pronounced. Nova Scotia also depends on federal transfers more heavily than many provinces, and the shift to per-capita calculations as well as the move to reduce the CHT escalator (the rate of growth of transfer payments) to 3 per cent will have a serious impact on the province's health care budget.

Given Nova Scotia's older demographic, cost pressures will also be experienced in the long-term-care and home-care sectors, as well as in pharmaceuticals. One small source of optimism is that Nova Scotia is a leader in moving away from fee-for-service payments to physicians. Given that a relatively large proportion of the province's physicians are paid at least partially through alternative (or academic) payment plans, there is a possibility that such payment systems can be used to develop more collaborative health care bodies that (at least in theory) provide better access with less cost. To a certain extent, however, there is a limit to what the province may be able to accomplish in isolation; and its prospects may depend more than ever on the wider intergovernmental context.

Chapter Four

Physical Infrastructure

Health care infrastructure includes physical assets such as buildings, land, equipment, and information technology (IT) systems. Provinces are generally responsible for the cost of this infrastructure: while Ottawa provided hospital construction grants for the provinces from the 1940s to the early 1960s, the terms of the 1957 Hospital Insurance and Diagnostic Services Act and the 1966 Medical Care Act provided federal health transfers only for hospital and physician services (although these transfers in practice are not conditional, but become part of provinces' general operating revenues). The federal government has provided funding to provinces to enhance specific infrastructure projects (such as diagnostic equipment or IT systems), but has chosen since the 1960s not to become involved in hospital construction projects.

This means that many of the large hospitals built in the middle of the twentieth century are coming close to the end of their natural lifespans. Two discrete policy issues have emerged because of this. The first is the deferring of the construction of major new hospitals. Capital costs for new hospitals tend to be quite high: the cost to replace a hospital in Halifax de novo, for example, was estimated at two billion dollars, approximately half of the province's entire health budget. Public-private funding has been considered as a means of financing new hospitals, but evidence regarding the long-term effectiveness of public-private partnerships (P3s) is quite limited (Klein et al., 2013). A second issue is the deferring of the maintenance of existing facilities. The maintenance of physical infrastructure is generally considered to be part of provinces' operating budgets rather than capital budgets, and thus tends to be "a common item on the hit list for operational cost reduction strategies" (Roberts & Samuelson, 2015, 17). This problem can be exacerbated in an economic environment of constrained economic growth, especially where lack of access to services becomes a politically contentious issue and facility maintenance has to compete with service provision for adequate funding. The pressure to defer maintenance becomes especially intense in provinces where governments have given priority to reducing or eliminating deficit spending.

There has been more transformation of physical infrastructure in rural Nova Scotia, where small emergency departments in eight regions have been replaced by "collaborative emergency centres" (CECs). While these facilities are not identical, the principle underlying these CECs is that they can be staffed during overnight hours by nonphysician health care professionals (usually nurses and paramedics), and that there is a close web of connectivity (by telephone, by ambulance, and by air ambulance) for cases requiring a level of care at regional or tertiary/quaternary care centres that CECs are unable to provide. Similarly, primary care reform in both rural and urban areas is focusing on the establishment of "collaborative care centres" (CCCs) to be staffed both by physicians and other health care professionals.

4.1 Hospital and other treatment facilities

"If funding stays at recent levels and available money is allocated as it currently is," stated Nova Scotia's auditor general in 2012, "Nova Scotia's hospital system cannot be adequately maintained and will continue to deteriorate" (Nova Scotia Office of the Auditor General, 2012c, 61). In the former Capital District Health Authority (CDHA) alone, for example, the auditor general's audit of equipment and buildings found that of the 13,000 pieces of medical equipment, 16.2 per cent were between 10 and 15 years old; 4.7 per cent were between 15 and 20 years old; and 5.3 per cent were more than 20 years old (ibid., 75). The consequences of depending on superannuated equipment became clear in 2015 when black flecks on sterilized equipment in the CDHA were found to have come from the highly corroded interiors of the sterilization equipment itself, which was almost 30 years old. At least 563 surgeries in the CDHA had to be postponed, and $500,000 had to be spent immediately to purchase new sterilizers. But the state of the buildings was the source of even greater concern. In September and December of 2015, high-pressure breaks in water pipes in an aging hospital within the Queen Elizabeth II Health Sciences Centre in downtown Halifax caused extensive and severe damage to three floors, requiring the evacuation of patients and the postponement of surgical procedures. Another burst pipe in August 2016 caused more flooding. The Auditor-General's Office had in 2012 noted the poor condition of many hospital buildings. As the construction industry usually recommends the replacement of facilities when the cost to repair exceeds the cost of replacement by 30 per cent, the 30 per cent figure was used as a benchmark to illustrate the condition of these buildings. Of the 53 facilities audited, in almost one-half of the cases (26) the cost to repair exceeded 30 per cent; 14 facilities exceeded 40 per cent; and four exceeded 50 per cent (ibid., 75–6).

Part of the problem with the maintenance of physical infrastructure rested in the lack of province-wide, long-term capital planning. Final decisions on capital planning were made by three committees at the provincial level: Infrastructure Repair and Renewal (for facility projects under $90,000); Infrastructure Management Repair and Renewal (for projects between $90,000 to $1 million); and Equipment (for all equipment requests). However, until 2013, district health authorities (DHAs) themselves had no input into developing the criteria for decision making or for the assessment of funding requests. Thus, health districts set their own priorities and developed their requests with very little understanding of the funding allocation process. Until 2015, Nova Scotia's 42 hospitals were distributed between nine DHAs, each operating under a year-by-year capital strategy. Moreover, many hospitals received only three-quarters of their total funding from DHAs, which meant that they depended on philanthropic foundations and local auxiliaries for up to a quarter of their funding. The fragmentation of capital planning was compounded by issues of jurisdictional authority: for example, hospitals were unable to engage in infrastructure-renewal projects such as energy-performance contracting because, under the existing Health Authorities Act, they were not legally permitted to incur debt without governor-in-council approval. At the same time, the Department of Health and Wellness (DHW) would not engage in such projects unilaterally due to its position that the DHAs were the legal owners of the facilities. As the province amalgamated the DHAs in 2015 and moved to implement multiyear capital planning, some of these issues were resolved, at least from a planning perspective. As the auditor general warned, however, "[t]he funding estimated for basic infrastructure repair and renewal over the coming decade will cost more than traditional funding amounts can cover. These estimates do not include the cost of all infrastructure or medical equipment, or costs for any new facilities" (Nova Scotia Office of the Auditor General, 2012b, 64–5). Thus the amalgamation of health

Figure 4.1 NSHA infrastructure funding gap, 2015–16

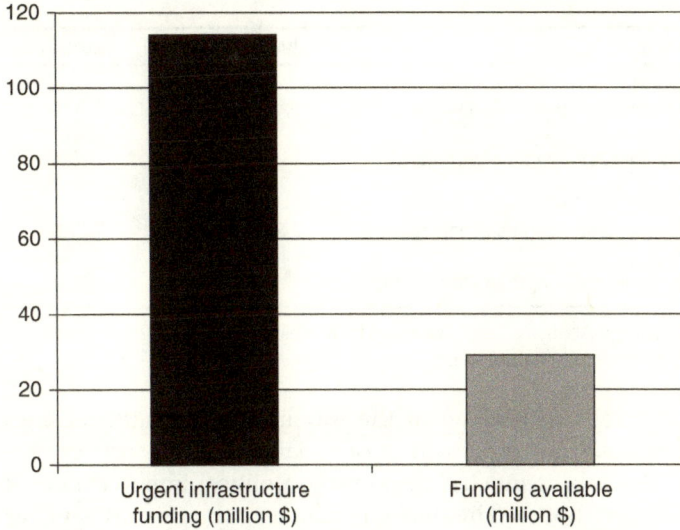

Source: Office of the Auditor General of Nova Scotia, June 2016 Audit Report, chapter 2
(http://oag-ns.ca/publications/2016), p. 35.

districts may be a useful streamlining of the decision-making process, but it does not address the shortfall in funding needed for health infrastructure to meet efficient working standards. As a 2016 audit noted, the gap between urgent infrastructure funding and available funding was considerable (Figure 4.1).

Notwithstanding the disquieting condition of health facilities in Nova Scotia, the health system itself has seen very positive changes in hospital-utilization rates. Acute inpatient hospitalization dropped from 114,953 in 1995–6 to 85,227 in 2010–11; standardized for age and sex, rates (per 100,000) dropped from 12,033 to 7,767 over the same period. Notably, the percentage change of –35.5 over the 15-year period was the most substantial drop across all Canadian provinces (CIHI, 2012b). By 2013–14 Nova Scotia's standardized hospitalization rate was very close to the national average (Table 4.1). Moreover, risk-adjusted 30-day readmission rates to acute care were (along with Alberta) the lowest in Canada in 2010–11 (CIHI, 2012a).However, length of stay in hospital was the highest in Canada (9.3 days): even adjusted for age, Nova Scotia still had one of the longest lengths of average acute hospital stay (along with Manitoba). The standardized cost of hospital stay in Nova Scotia, at $5,661, is slightly above the national average of $5,567 (CIHI, n.d.).

Table 4.1 Age-sex standardized acute inpatient hospitalization rates (per 100,000 population)

	2000–1	2010–11	2013–14
Nova Scotia			
Age and sex standardized hospitalization rate per 100,000	9,867	7,767	7,524
Age-standardized average length of stay (days)	7.7	8.5	8.4
Canada			
Age and sex standardized hospitalization rate per 100,000	9,363	7,635	7,596
Age-standardized average length of stay (days)	7.2	7.3	7.0

Source: CIHI Discharge Abstract Database/Hospital Morbidity Database (https://www.cihi.ca/en/hospital-morbidity-database).

The most notable re-thinking of the way in which health facilities are configured has been the creation of collaborative emergency centres (CECs). This was as much a response to political imperatives as it was to organizational ones. The public response to the Corpus Sanchez report on health care reform (submitted to the provincial government in December 2007; see chapter 2) was overwhelmingly negative, as rural communities worried that their small emergency departments would be shut down. The NDP capitalized on this sentiment during the 2009 election, promising that no rural emergency departments would be closed. This, however, was a difficult promise to honour, as small rural departments were costly and largely unnecessary. They also distorted the availability of primary care. For example, close to 90 per cent of visits to these small emergency departments involved conditions that could have been addressed in a clinic setting (in 2009–10, only 1.2 per cent of these cases were "life or limb threatening" or "severe," compared to 12.9 per cent of all cases presenting at the large Halifax emergency department). Most of these cases occurred during the day or evening: night visits averaged approximately one patient. But keeping doctors and nurses on duty during the night meant that they might not be able to work the next day, thereby reducing primary health care hours even further. This led to unpredictable closures of small emergency departments: across the province, emergency departments were closed for a total of 19,116 hours (equivalent to 795 days) in 2009–10 alone. The cost of keeping physicians on call for overnight emergencies was also substantial (approximately $350,000 to $700,000 per year per site) given the very small utilization rate (Nova Scotia, 2010a). Moreover, recruiters found it difficult to attract physicians to these smaller communities, partly because of the way in which doctors' work was structured.

Politically, then, the new NDP government was obliged to consider how to address the serious inefficiencies presented by rural emergency departments, without actually eliminating them. To this end this they commissioned an emergency physician, John Ross, to develop a plan for emergency care throughout the province, including the issues facing emergency departments in large hospitals. His reports were incorporated into *Better Care Sooner*, a 2010 document outlining a new approach to emergency care that, among other things, included the development of CECs for smaller communities (Nova Scotia, 2010b).

By 2015, eight CECs had been established. Formally, each CEC had three basic components: a primary health care team, urgent care capacity, and a protocol or plan for emergency care in conjunction with emergency health services (EHS) and DHAs. All CECs are slightly different, depending up on local need and available facilities and staffing. CECs generally are open for primary care for 12 hours a day, 7 days a week, and aim to accommodate same-day and next-day appointments (Nova Scotia, 2014b). This means that individuals can see a physician, nurse practitioner, or family practice nurse when they require attention, and especially for the management of chronic health conditions. Overnight, CECs are generally staffed by registered nurses and paramedics, who can confer by phone with an emergency physician if necessary. Given the ready accessibility of primary care appointments, the presentation of emergency cases at night is minimal (less than one individual per night, on average, with no patients at all 44 per cent of the time) (ibid. 29).

A 2014 consultant's report on the state of CECs was highly positive (Nova Scotia, 2014b). Given the ease of making primary care appointments in CECs, nonurgent (CTA 4–5) cases presenting in the emergency department during both the day and the night have dropped sharply. Unplanned day-to-day closures of rural emergency departments have also fallen significantly. Both patients and providers report satisfaction with the CEC model. There are some issues with care provided by CECs that still have to be sorted out: for example, laboratory and X-ray facilities are generally offered only during traditional office hours, which presents an obstacle for patients who have primary care visits scheduled in the evening. Primary and emergency care within some CEC facilities are too far apart physically, which can make it difficult for both providers and patients to move efficiently from one to the other. Same-day scheduling can mean that some patients will not see their regular physician, which can affect continuity of care, especially for those requiring close chronic-disease management. Overall, however, the CEC model is considered a clear success. Ironically, the CEC model has been so successful that it has made overnight emergency care almost unnecessary, even though it was the need to provide a new form of overnight emergency access that precipitated CECs in the first place. There is currently discussion about changing overnight access such that paramedics would respond on-site to any emergency call and, if required, would transport a patient to a regional hospital. This would allow CECs to close their overnight emergency departments altogether, though officials will no doubt gauge public response carefully before proceeding on this course.

Treatment facilities in Nova Scotia also include institutions designated for rehabilitation. This includes addiction rehabilitation (including treatment for prescription opiate addiction), physical rehabilitation, and vocational rehabilitation for mental health patients. Although a 2016 report noted that more than 42,000 Nova Scotians required help for addiction problems in 2014–15 (Laroche, 2017), fewer than 20 alcohol and drug rehabilitation centres are located in the province. Seven are detox facilities; seven are residential centres (two of which are specifically designated for indigenous clients); and the remainder are outpatient clinics. Most facilities are operated by the Nova Scotia Health Authority (NSHA); some are privately run. While there are formal standards for such provincial treatment facilities, these standards are voluntary. A 2012 audit performed by the auditor general found that there was little monitoring of these services by the DHW for compliance with provincial standards (Nova Scotia Office of the Auditor General, 2012a).

Physical rehabilitation is also under the jurisdiction of the NSHA, and treatment facilities are generally located within hospital settings. The Nova Scotia Rehabilitation Centre (NSRC) is by far the largest of these, and 43 per cent of the inpatients are from outside the Halifax Regional Municipality. The NSRC provides inpatient, outpatient, and outreach services in five principal areas: neuro and spinal-cord injury, acquired brain injury, musculoskeletal, assistive technology, and person-centred ambulatory care. There are three inpatient units at the NSRC: acquired brain injury, musculoskeletal, and neurology and spinal-cord injury.

The historical context of vocational rehabilitation services for mental health patients, as Fingard and Rutherford (2011) explain, is situated in the move from municipal to provincial funding for mental hospitals between 1958 and 1966. Given that federal hospital insurance did not cover psychiatric hospitals, "treatable" patients were moved to psychiatric wings of general hospitals, while chronic patients were dehospitalized. The latter were assisted financially through the new Canada Assistance Plan, which cost shared the care of deinstitutionalized mental patients. This resulted in the establishment of regional rehabilitation centres developed by private, nonprofit organizations such as the Canadian Mental Health Association. The largest of these rehabilitation centres is the LakeCity Employment Services Association in the Halifax Regional Municipality, which utilizes a model of "supportive employment" to facilitate the reengagement of patients into the community.

4.2 Long-term care facilities

Echoing the auditor general's concern that hospital facilities were unsustainable given existing funding patterns, the deputy minister of health and wellness in 2015 declared that "we are on a track that is not sustainable" in long-term care (Nova Scotia Hansard, 2015b). Nova Scotia spends over $800 million per annum on continuing care services. This amounts to approximately 20 per cent of the total health budget. The national per capita utilization of nursing home beds is 86 per every 1000 people over 75; in Nova Scotia it is 113 per 1000, with a goal to increase the number to 115 per 1000. In 2006, when Nova Scotia released its 10-year continuing-care strategy (*Continuing Care Strategy for Nova Scotia: Shaping the Future of Continuing Care* [Nova Scotia, 2006]), the number of individuals waiting for a long-term-care bed was 1,079 (Nova Scotia Office of the Auditor General, 2011, 99). Almost 10 years later, despite adding 1,018 new beds, the number of individuals waiting for a long-term bed had almost doubled to 2,126. Of these individuals awaiting bed placements, 1,940 were waiting at home and 186 were in hospital. This is despite a change in waitlist policy: as of March 2015, individuals who refused a nursing-home bed when one became available no longer had the option to defer the placement; rather, they would be removed from the waiting list altogether (although they would have the ability to be waitlisted again after 3 months). Prior to this change in policy, the waiting list was close to 2,500. In addition, since March 2015 an oversight committee has been charged with evaluating the wait list more scrupulously to ensure that those on the list for long-term care needed to be there (Nova Scotia Hansard, 2015b). In 2015, Nova Scotia had a total of 7,824 long-term care beds. The average wait time for a bed was 333 days in 2014–15 (up from 169 days in 2006–7), although this depends on the region and the facility (the range of wait times is between 30 days and one year). Equally problematically, the placement protocol for long-term beds is currently not based on need but rather on when one is placed on the list.

4.3 Diagnostic facilities

4.3.1 Laboratory services

Nova Scotia has a single government-run laboratory system. Each health zone within the NSHA has its own set of laboratory facilities, but the largest and most comprehensive clinical laboratory is located in the QEII Health Sciences Centre in Halifax (affiliated with Dalhousie's Department of Pathology and Laboratory Medicine), which provides specialized testing and diagnostic consultation for the entire province. The NSHA also operates blood-collection services, although the province does permit private blood-collection agencies as well (there are 76 independent blood collectors operating in the Halifax Regional Municipality alone). However, those working in the private collection agencies require no certification or licensing. This led to some concerns about quality assurance, as audits conducted by the former CDHA found that independent phlebotomy errors "averaged from 12–54 times higher" than those done by public blood-collection services (Capital District Health Authority, 2014c). In May 2014, the health authority announced that it would no longer accept blood samples from one of the independent companies (Atlantic Blood Collection).

4.3.2 Diagnostic imaging

The Auditor General's Office flagged the poor state of diagnostic equipment in both its 2007 and 2012 reports. Except for emergency purchases, noted the former, Nova Scotia had for years not funded capital equipment purchases, relying instead on hospital foundations and the federal Medical Equipment Fund (Nova Scotia's share of which amounted to $92.1 million) (Nova Scotia Office of the Auditor General, 2007, 10). By 2015–16 the province had budgeted $10,500,000 for "hospital equipment," although it is not clear if diagnostic imaging equipment is part of this allocation. Both the 2007 and 2012 reports highlighted the aging state of diagnostic equipment in the province, noting that the CDHA had even procured two ultrasound machines from a hospital in PEI that was disposing of them (ibid., 17). Using an industry standard of 10 years as an average lifespan for diagnostic imaging equipment, the auditor general observed that "[a]cross Canada, 4 per cent of CT scanners in use in 2005 were more than 10 years old, while at CDHA and CBDHA, 25 per cent were more than 10 years old. The two MRIs in use at CDHA were 10–12 years old as of January 1 2007, while only 6 per cent of the MRIs used in Canada were more than 10 years old" (ibid., 16). According to a 2015 audit of Canadian medical-imaging capacity, Nova Scotia had 21 CT scanners on 16 sites, 11 MRIs on 10 sites, seven SPECT on four sites, one PET-CT scanner, and nine SPECT-CTs on eight sites (Canadian Agency for Drugs and Technologies in Health, 2015).

Wait times for diagnostic tests are posted on the province's website. According to national benchmarks on wait times for diagnostic services, Nova Scotia's average wait time for CT scans (74 days) was the longest compared to five other provinces; MRI wait times were even longer (202 days) (CIHI, 2016c). There is much regional variability for both CT and MRI wait times, with those in the Halifax Regional Municipality often having to wait more than twice as long for services compared to those in some smaller communities. This may explain why Halifax also has a private diagnostic clinic, which was established in 2006 by two radiologists working in the former CDHA. The clinic, HealthView Medical Imaging, is part of the Canada Diagnostic Centres chain of clinics across Canada and in 2015 offered MRI scans for $795 (via a Sigma 1.5T LX), ultrasound services for $250 (via a Philips IU22), and bone densitometry for $140 (via a General Electric Lunar). These scans (in free-standing clinics) have been delisted by the province as publicly insured benefits, and the service has been used both by individuals paying out of pocket and by third-party insurers. A Fredericton company, Atlantic Medical Imaging, opened another private diagnostic facility in the Halifax Regional Municipality in January 2014. This facility boasted a state-of-the-art low-radiation scanner (Toshiba's Aquilion One) that provided ultrasounds for $396 and 640-slice CT scans for $683. But the business model for this company depended on securing public contracts, and the government made a decision to remain with its lower-resolution, publicly owned equipment. By May 2015, the business closed and was placed in receivership.

The existence of private diagnostic facilities has led the auditor general to raise concerns about conflicts of interest for medical staff involved in the establishment and operation of private facilities. The Nova Scotia College of Physicians and Surgeons has enacted by-laws referencing its conflict-of-interest guidelines. These guidelines stated that the terms of any agreement whereby a physician gains an ownership or proprietary interest in a facility should not

- be related to the past or expected volume of referrals of patients or other business from the member to the Facility;
- include any requirement that the physician make referrals to the Facility or otherwise generate professional business for the Facility as a condition for entering or continuing the agreement; or
- provide the physician with a return on investment directly attributable to the physician's volume of referrals to the Facility. (College of Physicians and Surgeons of Nova Scotia, 2013)

The Nova Scotia Health Authority also has enacted a general conflict of interest policy for all employees (Nova Scotia Health Authority, 2015b).

4.4 Public health facilities

Public health functions are supported by the Provincial Public Health Laboratory Network of Nova Scotia. A number of public health laboratories are located across the province, with the main hub of the network located at the QEII Health Sciences Centre in Halifax. In 2009, the Public Health Laboratory Network conducted an evaluation of lab capacity in Nova Scotia and concluded that the network possessed adequate capacity to assist in surveillance activities concerning notifiable diseases. The Auditor General's Office also reviewed the network's assessment in 2009 as part of its audit of pandemic preparedness in the province and found that the network did not have any evident capacity problems in the event of an outbreak scenario (Nova Scotia Office of the Auditor General, 2013).

4.5 Information and communications technology infrastructure

Information technology systems are increasingly seen as an essential foundation for safe, efficient, and cost-effective health care systems. To this end, Nova Scotia has been particularly concerned with the development of its electronic health infrastructure. Despite some of the problems noted above regarding the state of diagnostic equipment and buildings in the province's health care system, Nova Scotia's electronic health information system compares quite favourably with other provinces, both in terms of the types and level of services provided and in the interoperability of electronic record systems across the province. Beginning in 2002, Nova Scotia established a core set of electronic health care systems, including the Nova Scotia hospital Information System (NShIS), which served as the basis of its electronic health records (EHRs) network. The Picture Archiving Communication System (PACS), which provided electronic access to medical images such as scans and X-rays, was added in 2003; and electronic medical records (EMRs) were developed in 2005 through the Primary Health Care Information Management (PHIM) program, providing electronic record-keeping tools for primary health care professionals. Another cornerstone of the electronic health care information system is the development of a personal health record (PHR) system, which began as a pilot program in 2012. Tied into these core programs are more specialized electronic information systems such as the Patient Access Registry and Drug Information System (Figure 4.2). In 2006, Nova Scotia mandated Health Information Technology Services Nova Scotia (HITS-NS) to develop, manage, and lead the province's health IT infrastructure.

4.5.1 Core electronic information systems

The core electronic information systems include EHRs, which are secure electronic records of a patient's medical history that can be accessed by authorized health care providers throughout the province; EMRs, which are electronic records that replace the paper files of patient information held by a patient's health care provider; and personal health records (PHRs), which are electronic records of an individual's health information that are maintained by the patients themselves.

ELECTRONIC HEALTH RECORDS (EHRs)
The first step in establishing a comprehensive EHR system was the development of the **Nova Scotia Hospital Information System** (NShIS). Interfaced with more than 180 different types of diagnostic equipment, the NShIS was the first jurisdiction-wide multihospital implementation of this system in North America (Nova Scotia Office of the Auditor General, 2005). Evolving from the provincial Health Information Strategy that was articulated in the mid-1990s, the NShIS was initiated in March 2001, phased in in February 2002, and fully operational by April 2005. Developed at a cost of approximately $55 million, the goal of the program was to implement a system (the Meditech program) that could allow 34 hospitals across eight district health authorities efficiently to

Figure 4.2 Nova Scotia's electronic health information system

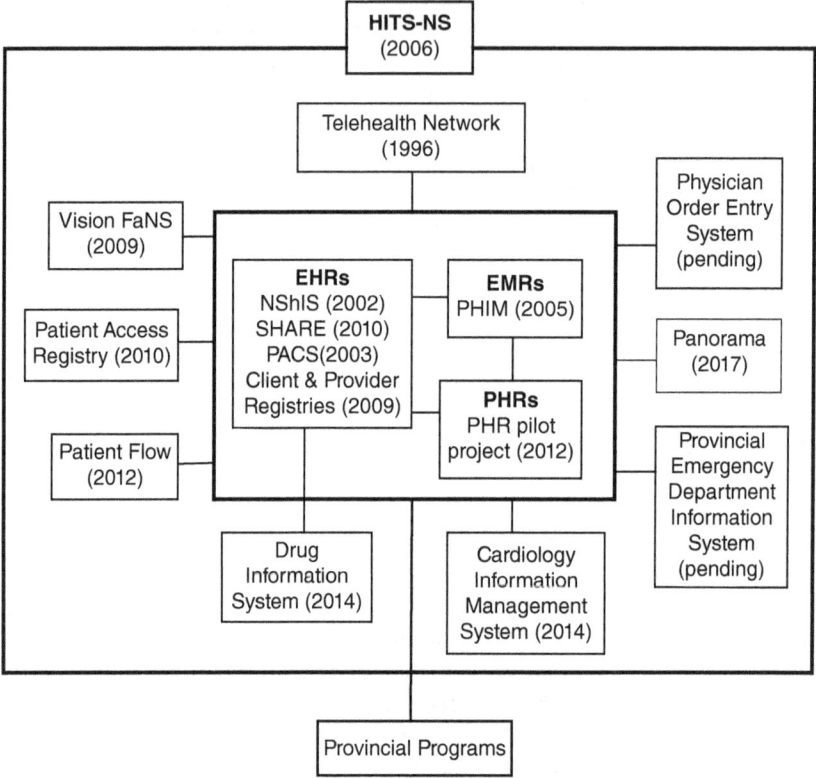

share clinical information. The ninth (and largest) DHA, the CDHA, did not possess a single information system but rather had selected the best electronic program ("best of breed" approach) for each particular function that was required. The remaining DHA, the IWK Children's Hospital, had a different but functionally similar system to that which was implemented in DHAs 1 to 8. Because of the need to extend interoperability to all DHAs, the province then applied to Canada Health Infoway to widen and deepen its electronic health record system (NShIS had been developed without Canada Health Infoway funding).

Having secured $19.2 million in funding from Canada Health Infoway, the province committed an additional $9.1 million to the development of the **Secure Health Access Record** (SHARE) project, which became operational in 2010. SHARE permitted hospitals across all DHAs to communicate with each other. The key components of SHARE were the **Client and Provider Registries,** which came on line in 2009, and the **Picture Archiving Communication System** (PACS), which allows health care professionals instantaneously to access images such as angiography, CT scans, X-rays, MRIs, and ultrasounds across the province. Because of the high level of interoperability achieved through the common utilization of the Meditech system across most DHAs, which encompassed 28 of the province's 34 acute care facilities and 1,457 of 2,755 inpatient beds (Power, 2009), the implementation of PACS was relatively quick and effective. Nova Scotia initiated PACS in 2003 and, by 2006, it became the second province to attain 100 per cent implementation of this system.

ELECTRONIC MEDICAL RECORDS (EMRS)

The second pillar of Nova Scotia's electronic health infrastructure is the system of Electronic Medical Records. The **Primary Health Care Information Management** (PHIM) program run by the DHW provides support to doctors, clinics, long-term facilities and others in facilitating the use of electronic medical records. In 2005, the DHW awarded Nightingale Informatix, an Ontario-based company, a contract to be the exclusive service provider for EMRs. Nova Scotia is the only province in which the health department itself has contracted directly with the vendor and sublicenses the program to physicians. By having one publicly supported EMR vendor and a single government-run laboratory system, Nova Scotia was able to achieve a relatively high level of interoperability fairly quickly. This was bolstered by a provincial incentive of $10,000 for each doctor using Nightingale software, a measure which increased interoperability but which left local vendors furious that they had been cut out of a lucrative market (Howe, 2013). Between 2008 and 2016, Nova Scotia spent $39 million in incentives to physicians to utilize EMRs, including one-time payments of $5,300 per physician to offset up-front costs, annual per-physician payments for ongoing education in EMRs, and additional annual payments of approximately $5,600 for using EMRs (Colbert, 2016). Nine hundred physicians in Nova Scotia were using EMRs by 2015 (Doctors Nova Scotia, 2015). By 2015, physicians could choose from three systems (Nightingale-on-Demand, Practimax, and QHR Accuro) that were eligible for provincial funding support (in 2016, Nightingale was acquired by Telus Health). Unfortunately, these three systems do not effectively communicate with each other, which limits their overall utility. And, in 2015 the DHW decided to pause the number of doctors who could use EMRs in provincial hospitals due to a concern that there was no "consistent approach" in the use of EMRs in hospitals (Tunney, 2015). The province embarked on a new EMR strategy in 2015 to address these issues.

The 2014 National Physician Survey gives a glimpse of the way in which some Nova Scotia physicians use EMRs (Table 4.2). According to the survey, 12.5 per cent of respondents were using paper records only, 56 per cent used a combination of paper and electronic records, and 31.4 per cent used electronic records exclusively (however, this is a weighted sample of 405 respondents, and may not be representative of Nova Scotia physicians as a whole).

PERSONAL HEALTH RECORDS (PHRS)

The third leg of the core triad of electronic record systems is the PHR system. PHRs are controlled by patients themselves. This system gives individuals access to their own health records (including lab and test results), but it also provides communication between patients and health care providers, allows individuals to request appointments as well as prescription renewals and refills online, and permits them to log any symptoms, side effects, or other self-monitoring data as they see fit. Individuals themselves set the privacy data and can control who is allowed to view the information in their records.

In 2012, a request for proposals was submitted by the province for a pilot project on PHRs, which was three-quarters funded by Canada Health Infoway. McKesson's RelayHealth system was selected for a two-year demonstration project. Thirty physicians in the CDHA each enrolled 100 patients, for an initial total of 3,000 participants, although the final number of participants was 6,000 patients from 35 practices. Because of the success of the pilot, the DHW launched a province-wide PHR project, MyHealthNS, in collaboration with Canada Health Infoway, which contributed $10 million to the $13.3 million project. This is the first province-wide PHR system in Canada. However, buy-in from physicians to the project is voluntary, and as of 2017 a long-term compensation plan for physicians using the PHR system was not finalized (under the pilot, physicians were not remunerated for email communication with patients). This may limit the scale of the system in practice. Another issue is the formal purchase of cloud-computing services: traditionally, the large financial outlay made by provinces in health care infrastructure was determined through capital spending allocations. But as provinces purchase cloud-based technology that requires neither hardware nor software, significant resources will have to be redistributed from

Table 4.2 Physician responses regarding EMR utilization, Nova Scotia, 2014

Question		Response (all physicians)
When you are capturing information about your patients, do you:	Use paper charts only	12.5%
	Use a combination of paper and electronic charts to enter and retrieve patient clinical notes	56.0%
	Use exclusively electronic records to enter/retrieve patient clinical notes	31.4%
What are your reasons for not using electronic records?	No suitable product for my practice	17.4%
	Too costly	21.4%
	Too time consuming	32.1%
	Privacy concerns	10.5%
	Reliability concerns	12.8%
	Lack of training	28.0%
	Planning to retire soon	32.4%
	Not available (e.g., hospital's decision)	35.5%
	Other reason	2.2%
	NR*	0.0%
How long have you been using electronic records in your practice?	Less than a year	7.7%
	1–2 years	16.2%
	3–4 years	23.1%
	5–6 years	13.8%
	Over 6 years	39.0%
	NR	0.0%
If you access electronic records in various locations, can you access the same electronic records from different settings?	Yes	80.5%
	Some	13.1%
	No	6.4%
	NR	0.0%
Which of the following barriers have you experienced in accessing electronic records?	No barriers	15.2%
	Compatibility with other electronic systems	56.3%
	Privacy	16.3%
	Hardware availability	21.1%
	Technical glitches/reliability	55.5%
	Lack of training	15.5%
	Firewalls/security issues	35.1%
	Other	9.3%
	NR	0.7%
Has the use of an electronic record in your practice provided any of the following clinical benefits?	Helped you access a patient's chart remotely	53.3%
	Potential medication error alert	28.3%
	Alerted you to critical lab values	52.2%
	Helped you order on-formulary drugs	26.6%
	Reminders for preventive care	22.3%
	Reminders for care that meets clinical guidelines	20.3%
	Better availability of lab results	77.0%
	Identified required lab tests	21.1%
	Facilitated communication with a patient	14.3%
	Other benefits	12.5%
	No clinical benefit	7.3%
	NR	1.2%

(Continued)

Table 4.2 Physician responses regarding EMR utilization, Nova Scotia, 2014 (Continued)

Question		Response (all physicians)
How has the quality of the patient care you provide changed since electronic records were implemented?	Much better	17.2%
	Better	41.8%
	No change	27.5%
	Worse	3.2%
	Much worse	0.7%
	Not sure	7.3%
	NR	2.2%
Since electronic records were implemented, the productivity at your medical practice has:	Greatly increased	6.3%
	Increased	30.9%
	Did not change	34.4%
	Decreased	17.7%
	Greatly decreased	2.4%
	Not sure	7.3%
	NR	0.9%
Rate your access to Electronic Health Records (EHRs)	Excellent	8.3%
	Satisfactory	44.7%
	Unsatisfactory	27.5%
	Not available in my jurisdiction	18.8%
	NR	0.8%

*NR = no response
Source: National Physician Survey, 2014, http://nationalphysiciansurvey.ca/result/2014-results
-nova-scotia/

capital funding into operational funding (Usher, Jayabarathan, Russell, & Mosher, n.d.).

4.5.2 Specialized electronic information systems

The longest-running component of Nova Scotia's electronic health communications system is the **Telehealth Network**. Established as a pilot project in 1996, the Telehealth Network is a video-conferencing system connecting health care facilities across the province. It was Canada's first province-wide Telehealth network. Given the high proportion of Nova Scotia's population that resides in nonurban areas, the network is quite useful in permitting patients to access specialized health care consultations without the need for long-distance travel. The network is also used for training and administrative purposes.

In 2009, the province purchased VISION software to provide a comprehensive and integrated **Food and Nutrition Services (FaNS)** system for the province. By 2009, the NShIS was operational, and the FaNS program was designed to interface with the Meditech, Meditech Magic, and Star information systems. The VISION FaNS system produces standardized inventory lists, nutrient information, diet codes, allergen lists, recipe names, and menu templates across all DHAs, allowing it effectively to provide menu options for each patient's requirements in a safe and cost-effective manner.

The **Patient Access Registry Nova Scotia** (PAR-NS) system is a centralized wait-time reporting system that was implemented in 2010 at a cost of approximately $12 million, cost shared with Canada Health Infoway. Wait times are calculated from the moment when booking requests made by surgeons are received by a hospital. This data is then collected and posted on the website of the DHW each quarter. An audit conducted by the Auditor-General's Office in 2014 found that "the website compares favourably with those in other provincial jurisdictions, in both ease of use and also, what is reported" (Nova Scotia Office of the Auditor General, 2014c, 51).

In 2012, Nova Scotia introduced a **patient flow** system purchased from Medworxx. This system was already in place in New Brunswick, British Columbia, and Alberta. The purpose of the program is, first, to establish a common framework for care coordination between regions and disciplines and, second, to identify barriers, delays, and interruptions to patient care In order to ensure bed utilization is as efficient as possible. Covering 39 acute-care facilities and 3,000 beds, the patient flow system assesses appropriate use of in-hospital stays and readiness for discharge. It examines flow-through problems such as ER overcrowding, surgery deferrals, and increasing off-service care. For example, the CDHA found that limited access to physiotherapy services at the Dartmouth General Hospital was acting as a barrier to efficient patient flow. The situation was improved by providing weekend physiotherapy services, allowing patients to be discharged earlier.

Another electronic system introduced by the province was the **Drug Information System** (DIS), which was announced in 2011 and which started coming onstream in 2014. The DIS is another shared-cost program between the province ($17.5 million) and Canada Health Infoway ($9.6 million), and it uses DeltaWare Systems' Medigent Drug Information System (also used in New Brunswick and Prince Edward Island). The purpose of the program is to provide electronic communication between prescribers, pharmacies, and other authorized health care professionals; to give health care providers immediate access to reliable information on pharmaceuticals; and to identify contraindications, potential medication conflicts, and individuals' allergies or adverse reactions to specific drugs. The system facilitates the tracking of narcotic prescriptions (such as oxycodone), which are responsible for most drug deaths in Nova Scotia (for a more detailed discussion of the Nova Scotia Prescription Monitoring Program, see chapter 6). The implementation of the DIS involved three streams: the first focused on community pharmacies and gradually linked pharmacies throughout the province into the DIS throughout 2013 and 2014. A record of all prescriptions entered by any pharmacy in the province is accessible to any other pharmacy in Nova Scotia (in this way, the system is able to identify individuals using multiple prescribers for the same drug). The second stream focuses on incorporating hospitals and community prescribers using the SHARE clinical portal; and the third, which began in 2015, concentrates on integrating the DIS with clinics' EMR systems (which will allow health care providers to e-prescribe directly to pharmacies, as well as giving physicians a complete record of each patient's prescription record).

Two other IT programs under development, the **Computerized Physician Order Entry** system and the **Emergency Department Information System**, were placed on hold in February 2015. Because of the impending amalgamation of the DHAs in April 2015, the DHW decided that the existing EHR systems of all units should be integrated more tightly before work continued on these programs. Under the NShIS, eight DHAs employed the Meditech system, while the IWK used Meditech Plus, and the CDHA used a number of different programs for various functions. In February 2015, the province issued a $1.25 million tender to develop an integrated record system for the new single health authority (the "One Person, One Record" initiative). This new system will replace SHARE, the current hospital-to-hospital communication system. It is envisioned that the new "One Person, One Record" system will also incorporate EMRs and PHRs. As part of a single integrated clinical information system, the two programs under development can potentially be implemented in a more efficient and less costly manner. The Computerized Physician Order Entry system is a three-year, $7.2 program that will permit doctors to order services such as pharmacy, laboratory, and radiology results digitally; and the Emergency Department Information system is a three-year, $8.3 million project that provides the DHW with statistics on emergency-department performance.

Finally, the Panorama program procured in 2017 permitted the province to move from a paper-based to an electronic public health information system. The first stage of implementation (2017–18) focused on vaccine inventory and immunization records; the second stage (2018–19) on communicable-disease investigation. Of the $7.1 million spent on the program, $4.2 was reimbursed by Canada Health Infoway.

4.6 Research and evaluation infrastructure

Nova Scotia is one of four provinces with no form of "Quality Health Council." Yet even where they exist, the functions of such quality councils are quite varied. Generally, these functions include gathering and evaluating population-health indicators; establishing benchmarks, assessing best practices, and suggesting revised protocols for specific programs; health technology assessment (HTA); the facilitation of health services research; and the coordination of information across jurisdictions. In Nova Scotia, as in many provinces, these functions are divided between discrete units. The **Population Health Assessment and Surveillance** (PHAS) unit within the DHW, for example, gathers and analyses both qualitative and quantitative data to support the province's public health programming. The **Research Methods Unit** in the NSHA provides a broad range of specific consulting services to researchers, including research design, data management, clinical trials design, and health technology assessment. There is no discrete HTA agency in Nova Scotia. Health research is also facilitated by the **Nova Scotia Health Research Foundation** (NSHRF), which was established in 2000. The primary objective of the NSHRF is to support health research in Nova Scotia, including medical, health policy, health outcomes, and health services research. Because Nova Scotia is a small jurisdiction with limited funding, an important function of NSHRF is to maximize leverage for researchers in the provinces (such as the provision of seed funding) in order to support their applications within the national health-research framework. It also provides specific services such as peer review, project management, and evaluation services. In addition, it facilitates collaboration and partnerships between health researchers in Nova Scotia, both within and between the public and private sectors.

In 2013, the **Maritime Strategy for Patient-Oriented Research Support Unit** (MSSU) was established under the aegis of the national Strategy for Patient Oriented Research (SPOR), an initiative developed under the guidance of the Canadian Institute of Health Research (CIHR). The MSSU involves three provincial governments (Nova Scotia, New Brunswick, and Prince Edward Island); health authorities from all three provinces; the Health Research Foundations in Nova Scotia and New Brunswick; maritime universities; and other stakeholder groups. Funding is on a one-to-one basis between the CIHR and provincial governments/health research foundations. One key objective of the MSSU is to coordinate and integrate health data, as well as access to this data, across the Maritime provinces to produce comprehensive research outcomes for patient-oriented care. The MSSU also offers consulting expertise and training support in patient-oriented care (Levy, McDonald, Krause, & Anderson, 2015). Another Nova Scotia component of the pan-Canadian SPOR network is Building Research for Integrated Primary Healthcare Nova Scotia (BRIC NS), which is a provincial research network focusing on the needs of those with complex health conditions.

But there remain serious gaps in Nova Scotia's research and evaluation infrastructure. There is, for example, little capacity to evaluate certain programs within the province. A 2006 document commissioned by the Department of Health, for example, noted that "[t]here is simply no capacity within the current system at a provincial and especially at a district level to undertake the type of coordination and development of infrastructure that is required to create an accurate picture of the outputs, impacts, and outcomes of Nova Scotia's primary health care system" (Nova Scotia Department of Health, 2006a, 22).

4.7 Summary

The poor state of physical infrastructure in Nova Scotia can be attributed to the convergence of four factors: a critical mass of older buildings; a consistently weak economy; high political demand for health care services; and deficit-conscious governments. The serious deterioration of health care facilities and equipment had been clearly noted by the province's auditor general in 2012 and by Accreditation Canada in 2013. Nonetheless, because of limited fiscal resources, consecutive governments have viewed infrastructure renewal with some trepidation. As noted in chapter three, Nova Scotia spends approximately the same amount on health care per person as do other Canadian provinces, which means that spending on services consumes a much higher proportion of Nova Scotia's GDP (e.g., almost double the health-spending-to-GDP ratio of Alberta). The focus on providing a similar level of services to that of other provinces despite a smaller fiscal capacity means that there is an increasing strain on infrastructure spending and a decreasing quality of physical infrastructure in the province.

The strain on infrastructure spending manifests itself in two ways. Deferred maintenance to save costs and meet budget targets is common because maintenance funds, which are part of the larger operating budget, can be restricted in the short term without much attention. In the longer term, however, the untenability of existing infrastructure becomes increasingly apparent, and replacement becomes more efficient, though more costly, than repair. The dynamics of capital renewal are slightly different. Few political administrations favour heavy public capital investment in large-scale projects that may not be completed until after their term in office. At the same time, few if any provincial governments have the capacity "to evaluate and manage capital structure, return models, and project finance in a sophisticated way that would mirror other large capital-intensive private industries" (Klein et al. 2013, 4). This includes P3s, which have the political advantage of reducing short-term public expenditure. Nova Scotia's own P3 experience with school construction underscored this point, as the auditor general noted that the province was incapable of providing effective oversight in the management of these contracts (Nova Scotia Office of the Auditor General, 2010b). Ontario's experience with P3 funding for hospitals was also problematic, and a 2014 audit noted that the Brampton Civic Hospital cost the province $200 million more than had it been financed and operated publically (Ontario Office of the Auditor General, 2008). Few theoretical analyses give unqualified support for P3 projects, especially in complex areas such as health care (McKee, Edwards, & Atun, 2006; Boardman, Siemiatycki, & Vining, 2016).

Given the widening fiscal capacity of provincial governments (Saillant, 2016) coupled with the public demand for nationally comparable health care services, health infrastructure in Nova Scotia faces serious competition for limited resources. The few innovative financing strategies available to provinces (such as P3s or equity offerings) require a level of fiscal and policy capacity that small provinces, and possibly even larger ones, do not enjoy. For this reason, there has been some discussion about the role of the federal government in reengaging in hospital infrastructure projects. This may be in the area of direct funding (following the historical precedent of the hospital construction grants) or in the development of collaborative intergovernmental ventures that could build capacity planning models, set benchmarks on expected returns of capital investment to guide capital decisions, and create a shared resource of skilled individuals and best practices in capital planning (Roberts & Samuelson, 2015; Klein et al., 2013).

A final problem with capital planning goes beyond issues of financing. Partly due to the legacy of the 1957 Hospital Insurance and Diag- nostic Services Act, which secured federal funding for hospital services, a systemic bias in Canadian health care exists towards hospital treatment. Patients who could be treated more effectively and economically in other environments are for a number of reasons treated in hospitals instead. This bias is exacerbated by the lack of a comprehensive program of pharmaceutical insurance across Canada, as patients, providers, and caregivers may resist discharge if individuals cannot afford their medication costs outside a hospital setting. But as the primary health care, long-term care, and mental health care systems continue to evolve, the role of hospitals may change substantially; and this shift in purpose for hospitals must be built into the planning process for new hospitals. Despite the muted policy debate over physical infrastructure (especially compared to the provision of health care services), it is nonetheless a highly complex policy issue involving short- and long-term planning, shifting utilization patterns, economic trade-offs, and potential intergovernmental negotiation.

Chapter Five

Health Human Resources

Access to physicians in Canada is a consistent political issue across all provinces (Fierlbeck, 2011). By international standards, Canada has a relatively low ratio of doctors at 2.6 per 1,000 population: in contrast, Australia has 3.5 physicians per 1,000 population, and Germany has 4.1 (OECD, 2017a). Moreover, with a rate of 7.9 graduating physicians per 100,000 population, Canada relies quite heavily on internationally trained medical graduates, (compared, e.g., to Ireland's rate of 21.9 per 100,000 population) (OECD, 2017b). Yet there is no clear association between avoidable mortality and overall physician supply (Watson & McGrail, 2009): the number of physicians per population is a very crude measure of access to primary health care, and health workforce planning is beginning to address other important variables.

One key factor is the distribution of the health workforce: while numbers of physicians have been increasing in Canada, they have been increasing more quickly in urban areas than in rural ones (CIHI, 2016d). An issue facing all provincial governments is how to attract medical personnel to rural areas. British Columbia's attempt to restrict the payment to physicians practising in areas without physician shortages led to a successful Charter challenge (Waldman) in 1997 that limited provinces' ability to use financial disincentives to encourage physicians to locate in underserviced areas. Positive financial incentives remain a major policy tool, but they are expensive. A more recent policy lever to influence the distribution of doctors has been the use of physician credentialing, in which physician privileges (e.g., to provide patient care in hospitals, or to order diagnostic tests) are withheld for new physicians in areas that are not underserviced.

The way in which physicians practise is another important variable in determining access to primary care. Physician supply planning assumes a relatively constant level of direct patient care hours over time, yet younger GPs tend to work fewer hours than previous generations (Evans & McGrail, 2008). Thus patient contact hours can actually diminish even as the number of practising physicians increases. One strategy undertaken to address gaps in access to primary care has been to develop collaborative care centres that incorporate a wider range of health care professionals working up to their scope of practice. Given that most medical conditions are associated with chronic illnesses (such as diabetes, heart disease, respiratory disease, and depression or anxiety), monitoring or even preventing chronic disease is a significant part of contemporary health care. To this end, increased patient contact as well as specialized care can be achieved through the use of family and advanced practice nurses, psychologists, nutritionists, and other health care professionals in conjunction with primary care physicians (Fiandt, 2006). Yet the development of this kind of collaborative practice is, in practice, quite complicated. As GPs are legally considered to be independent contractors rather than public employees, their clinics are generally established as small businesses and they must fund these other health care professionals directly. Successful collaborative primary care centres, especially in rural areas, may therefore require public assistance in terms of overhead, adjustments in fee schedules or billing practices, or regulatory changes to address scopes of practice or liability. And as IT systems provide more options for medical care, this administrative transformation may also have to incorporate infrastructure to accommodate telehealth, or payment options that include non-face-to-face contact. While team-based care can be more cost-efficient, there may thus be *increased* coordination costs, at least in the short term, related to the provision of such collaborative care centres.

The discussion concerning the optimal number and mix of health care personnel is also cross-cut with issues of economic sustainability and cost containment. As Deber (2008) points out, as governments respond to public complaints over access to health care services by increasing the number of medical graduates, the rate of health care spending increases. Indeed, expenditure per physician in Canada grew 34.3 per cent between 1999 and 2009 as medical-school enrolment was expanded across Canada (Evans, 2011, 20). Primary care reform must therefore address access to services in tandem with physician remuneration in order to avoid substantial increases in physician payment (Henry et al.,

2012). Leonard and Sweetman (2015), for example, document how larger federal health care transfers to the provinces through the early 2000s were responsible for significant increases in remuneration for doctors and nurses. While work intensity decreased slightly over this period, they observe, "the earnings of individual workers in these health professions increased at a substantially higher rate than experienced by the workforce outside the health sector" (157), leading to interesting questions about the role of the public sector in driving income inequality within Canada.

Another issue of note is the political relationship between physicians and provincial governments. One of the consequences of the adoption of public insurance systems across provinces was that physicians were able to negotiate a formal status as independent contractors rather than public employees. Nonetheless, there remained an element of quasi-corporatism in the relationship between doctors and the state, as the physicians' professional associations have worked quite closely with provincial authorities in setting fee codes, negotiating regulatory codes, and developing other policy initiatives. Because of their specialized expertise, physicians have in previous decades been able to maintain a great deal of political influence over health policy. As governments increasingly utilize information technology to mine their administrative databases, however, they have established a countervailing influence over health care providers that may potentially undermine the historical political influence of physicians and other health care providers (Tuohy, 2003). Health human resource strategies are thus highly complex issues interwoven with other political, economic, and normative issues; and promises of effortless resolution should be viewed with an element of scepticism.

5.1 Main workforce challenges

The primary barriers to efficient health human resource planning in Nova Scotia over several decades have been the lack of sufficiently detailed information on which to base long-term planning; the lack of coordination between jurisdictions; and the utilization of planning models that did not take into account the complexity of contemporary health care services. Current health human resource strategies in Nova Scotia have been driven by the recognition that provincial workforce challenges are influenced by larger national trends and that concerted cross-jurisdictional action was therefore essential in addressing them. In September 2000 Canada's first ministers explicitly agreed in principle to coordinate efforts on health human resources (HHR), and by 2001 many schemes addressing planning and recruitment began to take shape (the Atlantic provinces, for example, embarked on a thorough examination of education and training capacity and planning for the region).This was reinforced by the 10-Year Plan of 2004, which required as a condition of federal funding that provinces not only increase the supply of health care professionals but also set and publicize targets for training recruitment, and retention.

But such strategies required detailed baseline assessments of existing capacity for each health occupation in each province. To this end, Nova Scotia commissioned a detailed study of HHR (funded by Human Resources Development Canada), which was published in 2003. Yet the report was hampered by the fact that some necessary data simply did not exist. Nearly one half of the regulated health occupations, noted the study, were not routinely collecting the kind of age information that was essential for projecting outflows due to impending retirements. Neither did the province know the number of graduates who remained in the province one year following graduation, nor the number and type of health workers leaving the workforce, nor the reasons they did so (Human Resources Development Canada, 2003). Nonetheless, the report presented a quite detailed snapshot of the nature of HHR in the province, including useful comparisons to other provinces. As part of the 10-Year Plan's stipulation that provinces publicly identify their HHR strategies, Nova Scotia released an action plan on HHR in 2005. This strategy was drawn in very broad brushstrokes, however, and articulated expansive goals such as "improving Nova Scotia's capacity to plan for the optimal number, mix, and distribution of healthcare professionals" and "enhancing Nova Scotia's capacity to work with employers, educators, and others to develop a workforce that has the skills and competencies to provide safe, high quality care and work in innovative environments that respond to changing healthcare systems and population health needs." The 2007 Corpus Sanchez report on the province's health care system was unimpressed with the rhetoric, and noted that Nova Scotia's HHR infrastructure was "generally understaffed to meet even the most basic needs for transformation" (Nova Scotia, 2007a, 54). A more detailed attempt at HHR planning was conceived in 2008 under the Model of Care Initiative in Nova Scotia (MOCINS), which attempted to think about HHR challenges within the wider context of a model of care that was "patient-centred, of high quality, safe, and cost-effective" (Nova Scotia, 2010c, section 5.5). Nonetheless, driven by greater interregional financial disparity, easier interjurisdictional mobility, and wider demographic and organizational trends, HHR remains a difficult and complex policy area. Tables 5.1 and 5.2 indicate health workforce trends and density.

5.2 Physicians

Nova Scotia has, in recent years, enjoyed a comfortable physician-patient ratio in strict numerical terms; the problem has generally been more an issue of distribution and access. Because of its strategic geopolitical role, Nova Scotia saw an early influx of physicians and surgeons in the late eighteenth century (Marble, 1993), yet by the middle of the twentieth century the province's Medical Care Insurance Advisory Commission expressed the concern that "even now there are not enough doctors," and worried that the establishment of Medicare would exacerbate such shortages (Nova Scotia, 1967, 47). By 1989, however, these anxieties were reversed, and the Nova Scotia Royal Commission on Health Care stated quite bluntly that "there are too many physicians in Nova Scotia" (Nova Scotia, 1989, 22). Indeed, between 1970 and 1989 the supply of physicians had almost doubled, and remuneration increased markedly as well. By 1970 doctors in Nova Scotia had reached parity with the national average for physician remuneration; by 1986 their earnings were second only to Ontario physicians (ibid., 20).

Physician-specific health human resource planning was introduced in 2012 with the release of the document *Shaping Our Physician Workforce*, which used consultants' reports that profiled the existing physician workforce and developed a forecast for the number, type, and distribution of doctors over the 2012–21 period (Nova Scotia, 2012a). The report noted that the ratio of family physicians to specialists in the province was 42:58, which was a notable outlier from the national ratio of 50–55 per cent family physicians to 50–45 per cent specialists. Moreover, it pointed out that almost 60 per cent of the province's doctors practised within Halifax. (One must recognize, however, that the tertiary and quaternary services provided within Halifax also service New Brunswick, Prince Edward Island, and Newfoundland and Labrador, so the ratios would of necessity be skewed towards specialists practising in Halifax). At 780 Nova Scotians per specialist, the province by far enjoys the best patient-specialist ratio in Canada (Table 5.3). There is, however, little political capital in this fact, as shortages of specific specialists are continually highlighted in the media.

Table 5.1 Nova Scotia health workforce composition and trends, 2005–12

Profession	First year of regulation	Availability of training programs	2005	2008	2012	% change 2005–12	% female (2012)
Audiologists	NR	Y	53	62	69	30.2	72.5
Chiropractors	1972	N	98	114	132	34.7	47.0
Dental assistants	1976	Y	..	..	796	..	99.7
Dental hygienists	1973	Y	511	547	668	30.7	97.6
Dentists	1,891	Y	499	521	535	7.2	38.1
Dietitians	1,998	Y	436	457	528	21.1	98.5
Environmental public health professionals	NR	Y	62	51	77	24.2	..
Health information management professionals	NR	Y	129	164	170	31.8	95.3
Medical laboratory technologists	2004	Y	947	939	851	NC	85.3
Medical physicists	NR	N	10	11	14	40.0	14.3
Medical radiation technologists	1967	Y	522	545	558	NC	82.1
Midwives	2009	N	10	10	10	0.0	100.0
Occupational therapists	1972	Y	309	355	411	NC	92.7
Opticians	2005	N	..	..	247	..	..
Optometrists	1921	N	86	101	113	31.4	44.2
Paramedics	2005	Y	..	..	2,218	..	..
Pharmacists	1876	Y	1,065	1,093	1,209	NC	71.9
Physicians (excl. residents)	1828	Y	2,039	2,189	2,367	16.1	35.5
GPs			1,102	1,116	1,206	9.4	41.2
Specialists			937	1,073	1,161	23.9	29.8
Physiotherapists	1959	Y	529	570	584	NC	78.6
Psychologists	1981	Y	414	462	500	20.8	74.0
Regulated nurses			11,860	1,2121	1,2904	8.8	95.3
LPNs	1957	Y	3,127	3,250	3,652	16.8	95.1
NPs	2002	Y	41	82	135	229.3	96.3
RNs (incl. NPs)	1910	Y	8,733	8,871	9,252	5.9	96.4
Respiratory therapists	2007	Y	141	252	261	85.1	72.8
Social workers	1994	Y	1,531	1,639	1,821	18.9	..
Speech-language pathologists	NR	Y	171	192	221	29.2	98.2

..: information not available
NR: not regulated
NC: data is not comparable due to a change in data source and/or methodology between 2005 and 2012
Source: CIHI, Canada's Health Care Providers: Provincial Profiles 2012. Available at https://secure.cihi.ca/estore/productFamily.htm?locale=en&pf=PFC2500

Table 5.2 Health workforce density, Canada and Atlantic provinces, 2005 and 2012

Profession	Nova Scotia per 100,000 population		New Brunswick per 100,000 population		PEI per 100,000 population		Newfoundland per 100,000 population		Canada per 100,000 population	
	2005	2012	2005	2012	2005	2012	2005	2012	2005	2012
Audiologists	6	7	6	9	3	3	3	5	4	5
Chiropractors	10	14	8	6	6	5	10	12	22	24
Dental assistants	..	84	..	81	..	112	..	36	..	75
Dental hygienists	54	71	39	62	42	58	18	35	57	79
Dentists	53	57	40	44	45	51	33	36	58	61
Dietitians	46	56	43	44	46	45	28	34	25	30
Environmental public health professionals	7	8	6	7	6	8	4	5	4	5
Health information management professionals	14	18	14	18	12	16	8	20	10	14
Medical laboratory technologists	101	90	88	86	79	47	81	106	62	NG
Medical physicists	1	1	1	1	3	4	1	1	1	1
Medical radiation technologists	56	59	67	74	52	60	56	71	49	52
Midwives	1	1	NA	0	..	..	..	..	2	3
Occupational therapists	33	43	33	42	24	33	25	35	35	39
Opticians	..	26	..	29	..	22	..	18	..	21
Optometrists	9	12	13	15	13	14	8	11	12	15
Paramedics	..	234	..	148	..	103	..	155	..	109
Pharmacists	114	128	84	102	116	117	114	128	91	95
Physicians (excl. residents)	217	250	173	221	144	182	194	240	190	214
GPs	117	127	103	117	89	98	99	126	98	109
Specialists	100	123	71	104	55	84	95	114	93	106
Physiotherapists	56	62	57	63	36	51	39	44	49	53
Psychologists	44	53	35	44	20	23	38	38	45	48
Regulated nurses	1,264	1,363	1,360	1,487	1,486	1,503	1,599	1,624	991	1,043
LPNs	333	386	352	388	439	438	526	434	201	252
NPs	4	14	3	X	NA	3	13	23	3	9
RNs (incl. NPs)	931	977	1,008	1,099	1,046	1,066	1,072	1,190	776	775
Respiratory therapists	15	28	30	54	12	21	14	25	24	31
Social workers	153	192	196	224	144	185	207	286	92	119
Speech-language pathologists	18	23	23	29	18	24	19	23	20	25

..: information not available
NG: data was not generated because data was unavailable from one or more provinces
X: value suppressed in accordance with CIHI's privacy policy
Source: CIHI, Canada's Health Care Providers: Provincial Profiles 2012. Available at
https://secure.cihi.ca/estore/productFamily.htm?locale=en&pf=PFC2500

Table 5.3 Population per physician, Atlantic provinces and Canada, 2013

	NS	NB	PEI	NL	Canada
All physicians	382	441	526	415	455
GP	749	820	943	792	897
Specialist	780	951	780	869	923

Source: CMA, Canadian Physician Statistics 2015.

Despite positive overall ratios, anxiety over physician staffing is driven by relatively high levels of physician outmigration (Table 5.4) and low levels of remuneration (Figure 5.1). In 2008–9 Nova Scotia's physician compensation was low but still surpassed New Brunswick and Quebec; by 2012–13 Nova Scotia's level of average clinical payment to physicians had fallen to the bottom of all provinces. This, to some degree, was driven by the contract cycle of fee negotiation in Nova Scotia, as the five-year Master Agreement contract was ratified in 2005 and then extended until 2015. Because no new base increases had been introduced over this period, causing physician salaries to fall relative to other provinces where contract agreements were ratified, the negotiations between physicians and province for a new Master Agreement proved to be quite difficult. In 2015, the province spent 19.5 per cent of its health care budget on physician services and programs (Table 5.5); though, as a point of reference, physician services in 1948 (prior to the Medical Care Act) accounted for 39.8 per cent of the province's health care budget (Nova Scotia, 1950, 110).

Dalhousie Medical School is a significant source of physician development for the province (47 per cent of practising physicians in Nova Scotia are Dalhousie graduates). The province estimates that approximately a third of current physicians will retire by 2021, which is in line with the national profile (Nova Scotia, 2012a, 4). Thirty-seven per cent of all physicians are female, but the numbers differ considerably for different age cohorts: 16.3 per cent of physicians over 65 are female, compared to 55.5 per cent of those who are under 35 (CMA, 2015). Nova Scotia also relies heavily on foreign-trained doctors: in 2015, only 71.4 per cent of the province's physicians graduated from a Canadian university (ibid.). This reliance has been especially pronounced in recent years, as international medical graduates filled almost 40 per cent of vacancies and new positions between 2002 and 2012 (Nova Scotia Department of Health and Wellness, 2012a).

Recruitment and retention strategies are thus important in securing physicians for rural areas. For those who have completed medical

Figure 5.1 Average gross clinical payments to physicians, 2008–9 and 2012–13 ($)

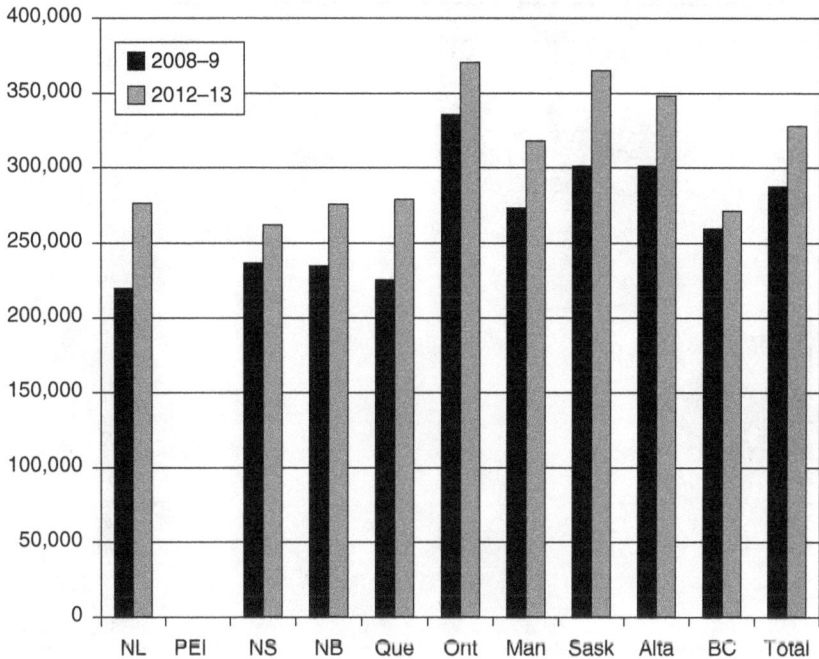

*Due to the significant skewing effect on physician counts and their associated payments caused by visiting specialists and locums, a comparable average physician payment is not included at the request of PEI.
Source: CIHI, National Physicians Database 2012.

training, the Debt Assistance Program offers between $20,000 to $50,000 in debt assistance to doctors in rural Nova Scotia. For current medical residents and fourth-year students, return-of-service bursaries of up to $60,000 are available to those willing to practise in rural Nova Scotia for at least three years. Since 2014, tuition relief of up to $120,000 has also been available for those establishing a new full-time practice in selected locations. Physicians relocating outside of metro Halifax are eligible for a $5,000 relocation allowance. The 2008–15 Master Agreement provided for a number of other measures to attract physicians to rural areas, including an expansion of the rural locum program, alternative funding arrangements (see chapter 3), access to electronic medical records, and "competitive compensation rates." Broader program changes have also been made to encourage rural practise, including a summer preceptor program in rural areas for first and second year medical students, a mentorship program for new graduates working in rural

Table 5.4 Net interprovincial migration by physicians, Atlantic provinces, 1990–2013

	NS	NB	PEI	NL
1990	−19	−11	3	−52
1991	−8	−3	0	−44
1992	−2	−7	2	−40
1993	−11	−5	2	−23
1994	−36	17	6	−37
1995	−2	16	0	−34
1996	6	7	0	−23
1997	24	9	1	−28
1998	12	1	6	−40
1999	1	4	10	−40
2000	−4	−11	−3	−50
2001	−22	6	6	−40
2002	−15	−2	2	−58
2003	−4	4	3	−41
2004	1	−11	8	−46
2005	−3	−13	0	−28
2006	−25	−4	0	−18
2007	6	11	2	−35
2008	−11	−9	3	−15
2009	−22	−10	2	−36
2010	−26	12	−3	−20
2011	−2	−8	8	−19
2012	−9	−14	−4	−18
2013	−15	−8	−7	−44

Source: CMA, Canadian Physician Statistics 2015.

Table 5.5 Spending on physician services in Nova Scotia, 2016–17 estimate ($ thousands)

Fee For Service	303,824
Radiology/pathology	61,694
Academic funding plans	215,738
Alternative payment plans	42,491
Emergency departments	59,397
Physician residents	32,655
Other master agreement initiatives	35,385
Facility on call	12,225
Physician services – other programs	45,056
Total	808,465

Source: http://www.novascotia.ca/finance/site-finance/media/finance/budget2016
/Estimates-and-Supplementary-Detail.pdf

areas, and the development of more collaborative interdisciplinary care teams in underserviced areas (Nova Scotia, 2014c). From 2005 to 2015, the College of Physicians and Surgeons of Nova Scotia offered a Clinician Assessment for Practice Program (CAPP), which supported international medical graduates with a special provisional licence to practise under supervision in rural areas. After one year of supervised practise, a physician could take a national-level family practice examination in order to become fully qualified. This program also required successful applicants to work in underserviced areas of the province. While the program was able to fill approximately 45 positions over 10 years of operation, it was a very expensive program and had a low retention rate. CAPP was cancelled in 2015 and will be superseded by a program aligned with national assessments organized by the Medical Council of Canada and the Royal College of Physicians and Surgeons of Canada.

5.3 Nurses

When the Liberal government came to power in 2013, briefing documents noted that the province could face a shortage of 800 nurses within 5 years if no steps were taken to address the trend. By 2015, 185 acute- and long-term-care nursing positions throughout Nova Scotia remained vacant. Between 2013 and 2015, acrimonious labour strife informed the relationship between nurses' unions and the province, and pension changes made retirement an attractive financial option for senior nurses. As in the rest of Canada, the average age of registered nurses (who comprise approximately three-quarters of the regulated nursing profession) continues to increase: in 2011, the average age for RNs in NS was 46.9 years, compared to an average of 45.3 across Canada (Table 5.6). RNs in the underserviced rural areas tend on average to be older than those in urban areas.

Yet, since the first nursing strategy was released in 2001, there have been notable successes in developing a sustainable nursing workforce in the province. In 2001, Nova Scotia retained just 53 per cent of its nursing graduates; by 2014 this figure had increased to 90 per cent. The first nursing strategy (2001–6) committed $60 million to stabilizing the nursing workforce "by improving the quality of life for nurses, keeping experienced nurses in the system, and enhancing recruitment efforts" (Nova Scotia, 2007b,1; see also Nova Scotia Department of Health, 2007). The second cycle (2007–14) focused on making better use of the nursing workforce, increasing the retention of nurses, and improving

Table 5.6 Regulated nursing workforce profile, Nova Scotia, 2011

		RNs			LPNs			All Regulated Nurses		
		#	%	Canada %	#	%	Canada %	Total	%	Canada %
Employed in nursing workforce		9285	–	–	3710	–	–	12995	–	–
per 100,000 population		982	–	–	392	–	–	1374	–	–
Sex	Male	408	4.4	6.6	183	4.9	7.7	591	4.5	7.1
	Female	8877	95.6	93.4	3527	95.1	92.3	12404	95.5	92.9
Average age	Years	46.9		–	44.6		–	45.3		–
Age breakdown	< 30 years	909	9.8	12.1	419	11.3	16.9	1328	10.2	13.2
	30–4 years	691	7.4	10.3	388	10.5	11.8	1079	8.3	10.6
	35–9 years	815	8.8	10.9	460	12.4	11.9	1275	9.8	11.1
	40–4 years	1048	11.3	12.2	510	13.7	12.8	1558	12.0	12.3
	45–9 years	1596	17.2	14.2	559	15.1	13.4	2155	16.6	14.1
	50–4 years	1592	17.1	14.4	577	15.6	13.6	2169	16.7	14.2
	55–9 years	1475	15.9	14.0	433	11.7	11.2	1908	14.7	13.3
	60+ years	1159	12.5	11.9	364	9.8	8.3	1523	11.7	11.1
Employment status	Full-time	6005	64.7	58.6	1843	51.9	51.1	7848	61.1	56.9
	Part-time	2224	24.0	29.2	970	27.3	27.3	3194	24.9	30.4
	Casual	1056	11.4	12.1	738	20.8	20.8	1794	14.0	12.6
	Employed; status unknown	0	–		159	–		159	–	–
Place of work	Hospital	6137	66.2	61.6	1781	49.0	42.9	7918	61.3	57.0
	Community health agency	980	10.6	13.3	499	13.7	9.5	1479	11.5	12.7
	Nursing home /LTC facility	1091	11.8	10.0	1254	34.5	39.0	2345	18.2	16.9
	Other place of work	1068	11.5	15.1	100	2.8	8.2	1168	9.0	13.5
Area of responsibility	Direct care	8216	88.5	89.0	3652	99.0	97.6	11868	91.5	91.1
	Admin/education/research	1069	11.5	11.0	37	1.0	2.4	1106	8.5	8.9
Position	Managerial	964	10.4	6.9	87	2.4	1.6	1051	8.1	5.6
	Staff/community health nurse	7075	76.3	76.9	3436	93.1	91.3	10511	81.1	80.4
	Other positions	1238	13.3	16.2	166	4.5	7.1	1404	10.8	14.0
Highest education level in nursing	Diploma	4812	51.8	57.3	3710	100.0	100.0	8522	65.6	67.8
	Baccalaureate	4113	44.3	38.8	–	–	–	4113	31.7	29.3
	Master's/Doctorate	360	3.9	3.9	–	–	–	360	2.8	2.9
Location of graduation	Canada	8981	96.7	91.4	3669	98.9	97.5	12650	97.3	92.8
	International	304	3.3	8.6	41	1.1	2.5	345	2.7	7.2

the flow of nurses entering into the workforce. During this period, and in conjunction with a series of pilot projects undertaken by the Canadian Federation of Nurses Unions (under the aegis of Health Canada), Nova Scotia established the Research to Action project on nursing HHR strategies. Between 2009 and 2011, the Nova Scotia Nurses' Union, the Department of Health, the DHAs, nursing schools and other groups collaborated on the development of three objectives: implementing a coordinated approach to new-nursing-graduate hiring across the province; developing evidence-based guidelines for orientation and transition programs for nurses; and cultivating a mentorship program between senior and junior nurses. First-year nursing seats at Nova Scotia's universities increased from 306 in 2001 to 401 in 2014. The 2015 nursing strategy was, to a large extent, an attempt to fine-tune existing training, recruitment, and retention strategies. To meet shortages in specialty areas, more training was targeted for intensive care, mental health, pre- and post-op care, and operating room nursing. A fast-track program was introduced that recognized existing science qualifications, allowing students to graduate in 2 rather than 4 years; and graduations are now staggered to allow the health care system more easily to hire graduates throughout the year. Recruitment efforts even more assiduously target areas with the greatest need; and more attention has been placed on optimizing scopes of practice (Nova Scotia has the highest number of licensed practical nurses [LPNs], at 392 per 100,000 population, compared to the national average of 246 per 100,000).

One significant component of the nursing workforce is the nurse practitioner. Also referred to as advanced-practice nurses, nurse practitioners are experienced nurses with additional nursing education and clinical competencies, allowing them to diagnose and treat acute and chronic illnesses, disorders, and injuries within clearly defined areas. Provincially, their scope of practice includes ordering and interpreting laboratory and diagnostic tests, and prescribing and reordering medications, including monitored drugs (such as narcotics). In Nova Scotia, the employment of nurse practitioners increased a remarkable 229.3 per cent between 2005 and 2012, so that by 2012 there were 14 nurse practitioners per 100,000 population in the province (compared to a national ratio of 9 per 100,000). Nurse practitioners were an essential element for the HHR strategy for underserviced areas, and by 2016 the registry listed 147 nurse practitioners with active licences. There is nonetheless a concern that nurse practitioners are currently underutilized in the province: none of the 15 nurse practitioners who graduated in the province in May 2015, for example, found employment as a nurse practitioner after graduation (Gorman, 2016a). However, as part of the plan to move Nova Scotia physicians to collaborative primary care models (see chapter 6), nurse practitioners may increasingly be replacing doctors in walk-in clinics around the province (Gorman, 2016a).

5.4 Other health care professionals

5.4.1 Paramedics

Nova Scotia has been remarkably innovative in the ways it has used para-medicine in the delivery of health care within the province. Paramedics play a major role beyond emergency medicine in Nova Scotia. They were used in a pilot program in 2001 in the remote communities of Long and Brier Islands, where the lack of physicians led to a paramedic- and nurse-based primary care program. In the first phase of this program, paramedics provided 24/7 ambulatory care to the residents of these communities. This was followed by a second phase, in which paramedic services expanded to clinic roles and the delivery of nonemergency ser-vices, and a third phase in which nonemergency services were provided by a nurse practitioner, complex care was provided by paramedics, and preventive health care programs were provided by a health care team. This model served as the basis for the collaborative emergency centres established in 2011, in which nurses and paramedics staff clinics between the hours of 8 p.m. and 8 a.m. (see chapter 4).

Another notable utilization of paramedic services has been the Extended Care Paramedic Program that was established in 2011. This program focused on nursing homes in the Halifax region and desig-nated specially trained paramedics to work in nursing homes between the hours of 9 a.m. and 9 p.m., when most of the transfers from nurs-ing homes to emergency departments occur. Paramedics can treat minor cases (such as suturing small cuts) immediately, and have also been trained to do routine blood work. During the two-year pilot pro-gram, 73.5 per cent of patients treated were attended to in the nurs-ing homes. In more complex cases, a new model for the delivery of paramedic care has been developed that focuses on "slowing the pace of the call and increased collaboration with LTC physicians, staff, patient, and family" (Jensen, Travers, Marshall, Leadlay, & Carter, 2014, 90). In this model, paramedics establish a care plan with online physicians, and when the patient arrives at the hospital, he or she is met with a medical team that has the treatment plan in hand. This leads to a much quicker turnaround time for patients and minimizes time spent waiting for treatment in an emergency ward. The successful experience of geriatric-specific paramedics has, in turn, led to the utilization of paramedics in palliative care. As of May 2015, all paramedics in Nova Scotia (and Prince Edward Island) were trained to offer assistance with palliative symptom management (including pain, breathlessness, fear, and anxiety) in patients' homes. Paramedics have been trained to perform triage in emergency departments. Nova Scotia has also been the first province to offer training to paramedics designed specifically to treat mental health issues. From November 2015, paramedics learned how to identify signs and symptoms of mental illness, how to respond to individuals in a mental health crisis, and how to ensure patients find the appropriate care to manage their mental health.

Despite the success at using paramedics more widely within the health care system, there are obstacles to this strategy. One is staffing. As with other health care professionals, there is a shortage of paramedics, and especially advanced-care paramedics (ACPs) in Canada. Paramedics in Nova Scotia receive training through the privately-run Medavie HealthEd, a business that consolidated two professional training schools (the Maritime School of Paramedicine and the Atlantic Paramedic Academy) in 2012. However, pay levels in the Maritimes remain low: an advanced-care paramedic may earn $62,000 in Nova Scotia after 5 years of services; in other provinces, the equivalent salary might be $80,000 to $90,000 or above. Some provinces actively recruit ACPs from the Maritimes to meet their own staffing shortages: the Ontario Paramedic Association, for example, observes that "there is a much higher percentage of non-Ontario trained paramedics from [ACP level] accredited programs [working in Ontario]. The east coast (Nova Scotia, New Brunswick, Prince Edward Island) is the primary source of these paramedics" (Pike & Gibbons, n.d.). The second potential issue is the private for-profit nature of paramedic training and delivery. Unlike some provinces, paramedic training is run by private training facilities (with tuition for basic training costing around $15,000) rather than by public educational institutions. The training institution is owned and controlled by the same company that provides emergency health services for the province. To the extent that health care is being increasingly provided by private contractors, there is some concern that this may result in the creeping privatization of provincial health care.

Table 5.7 Summary of pharmacists' expanded scope of practice across Canada, 2015

Expanded Scope	BC	AB	SK	MB	ON	QC	NB	NS	PEI	NL	NWT	YT	NU
Provide emergency prescription refills	Y	Y	Y	Y	Y	Y	Y	Y	Y	Y	Y	N	N
Renew/extend prescriptions	Y	Y	Y	Y	Y	Y	Y	Y	Y	Y	Y	N	N
Change drug dosage/ formulation	Y	Y	Y	Y	Y	Y	Y	Y	Y	Y	N	N	N
Make therapeutic substitution	Y	Y	Y	N	N	Y	Y	Y	Y	Y	N	N	N
Prescribe for minor ailments/conditions	N	Y	Y	Y	N	Y	Y	Y	Y	P	N	N	N
Initiate prescription drug therapy	N	Y	Y	Y	Y	Y	Y	Y	Y	N	N	N	N
Order and interpret lab tests	N	Y	P	Y	P	Y	P	Y	P	N	N	N	N
Administer a drug by injection	Y	Y	P	Y	Y	N	Y	Y	Y	Y	N	N	N
Regulated pharmacy technicians	Y	Y	P	P	Y	N	Y	Y	Y	Y	N	N	N

Y = yes; N = no; P = pending
Source: Canadian Pharmacists Association (http://www.pharmacists.ca/cpha-ca/assets/File/news
-events/ExpandedScopeChart_June2015_EN.pdf).

5.4.2 Pharmacists

As with nurse practitioners and paramedics, Nova Scotia has a significantly higher proportion of pharmacists (128 per 100,000 population in 2012) compared to the national average (95 per 100,000). At the same time, given a larger older population and higher levels of chronic disease in the province, pharmacists likely have a relatively higher workload per person. Geographical access to pharmacies is reasonably good in the province, with three-quarters of the population living within 5 kilometres of at least one location, and almost all of the population living within 30 kilometres (Law et al., 2013). Internationally, Canada has been relatively successful in making advances in involving community pharmacists in the prevention and management of chronic diseases (Mossialos et al., 2015; see Figure 1); within Canada, Nova Scotia pharmacists have among the widest scopes of practice in the country (Table 5.7).

In 2013, Nova Scotia pharmacists were given the authority to give vaccinations, as well as to order and interpret diagnostic tests necessary to manage patients' drug therapy (e.g., ordering blood tests needed to determine the dose of blood thinners). The fee schedule set each vaccination at $11.50, increasing $0.25 annually for 3 years. In 2010, the province was among the first to pass legislation approving prescribing for minor ailments by pharmacists. A "minor ailment" pilot program sponsored by the Pharmacy Association of Nova Scotia, concluded in 2013, permitted pharmacists to prescribe treatments for 31 minor ailments. Patients could then receive prescriptions for these conditions without having to consult a medical doctor. However, as patients were required to pay out of pocket for these consultations, there was relatively little utilization of this program. Because of this, a new one-year program began in May 2015 that reimbursed pharmacists for the cost of assessing Pharmacare users for three common minor ailments (allergic rhinitis, cold sores, and some skin conditions). The purpose of this pilot was to determine whether permitting patients with minor ailments to access pharmacists for treatment of such conditions could redirect such patients away from GP and emergency-room visits, thus saving health care dollars and providing better access for patients (consultations with pharmacists in 2015 were billed at $20, compared to $31 for a physician visit).

In September 2014, Nova Scotia piloted the Bloom Program, a 27-month program focusing on the use of community pharmacists to meet the mental health needs of individuals in the community. The program focuses on individuals with "a diagnosed mental illness or addiction causing functional impairment and a current medication therapy issue" (Bloom Program, n.d.). The Bloom Program was grounded on the observation that community pharmacists have regular interactions with these individuals and could be used as part of a support system for them. Moreover, pharmacists are among the most accessible health care providers and are located even in rural and remote regions in the province. After a private assessment session by a pharmacist, those individuals interested in participating give consent to share their confidential information with other individuals (e.g., GP, family member); these people can be contacted by the pharmacist if necessary. The pharmacist then monitors the progress of the patient either through regularly scheduled and on-demand interaction (in person or by telephone), accessed on weekends and evenings as well as weekdays. Some pharmacists even make house calls.

The evaluation report of the Bloom Program was highly positive. Eighty-nine per cent of the patients in the program rated it as "excellent to very good," and 92 per cent indicated that they would recommend the program to others (Nova Scotia Department of Health and Wellness, 2016a, ix). The program was especially notable regarding two of its key objectives. First, four in five medication issues of patients in the program (such as unresolved symptoms or impaired functioning, adverse effects, overmedication, or dependence) were "fully resolved or improved" (ibid., vii). Second, patients became better able to navigate the health care system and to access other services in their community:

> 61% of patients reported that their pharmacist helped them access other mental health services; 42% were helped to access services for their physical health; 25% were helped to access addictions care; and 47% were assisted in finding other services and supports in their community. Almost three of every four patients surveyed (72%) reported being more aware of community resources and 47% were able to access them faster than previously. (ibid., viii)

Given the success of the pilot period, the province has decided to continue funding the program under the purview of the Nova Scotia Health Authority.

5.4.3 Midwives

In contrast to other health care professionals in the province, midwives are relatively scarce. As of 2015, 15 individuals held membership in the Association of Nova Scotia Midwives: of these, only nine were practising. Publicly funded midwifery services are offered in three areas throughout the province (the IWK in Halifax; Guysborough and Antigonish; and Lunenburg and Queens County). Midwives who work in these funded sites use the local hospital that has obstetrical services (St. Martha's Regional Hospital in Antigonish, South Shore Regional Hospital in Bridgewater, and the IWK Health Centre in Halifax). While midwives played an important role in early eighteenth-century Halifax, public funding for midwives in Halifax was eliminated by 1761 and wasn't resumed until 2009. A report on the regulation and implementation of midwives in Nova Scotia had, in 1999, recommended that midwifery be legally recognized as an autonomous, self-regulated profession and included as an insured service. This legislation, however, was put on hold as the low number of midwives in the province (four) presented procedural difficulties in the disciplinary process required by self-regulated status. By 2006, however, the Midwifery Act was passed, and supporting regulation (including the establishment of a midwifery regulatory council) was in place by 2009. Three DHAs expressed an interest in the midwifery program, and seven full time positions were allocated between them.

The program was short-lived in Halifax, however, where four midwives at the IWK hospital had been hired to fill three FTE positions. By December 2010 the IWK midwifery program was suspended when three of the midwives resigned and the fourth went on leave. This has largely been attributed to the clash between an institution where the dominant ethos was one focused on high-risk care, and a profession used to providing care autonomously in a home setting for low-risk women. However, other issues also contribute to the difficulties that Nova Scotia–regulated midwives face. One of the primary issues is the employment model in the funded sites. According to the Canadian Midwifery Regulators Council (2016), there are a variety of models in Canada, with only a few being employer/employee models (Saskatchewan, Manitoba, Northwest Territories). The majority of midwives in Canada practise as independent contractors. The independent-contractor model allows midwives to have hospital privileges and to work within their scope of practice. They are primarily accountable to their regulatory body rather than to their employer's policies and procedures.

A 2011 assessment of the midwifery program stated that "midwifery cannot long survive in its present state. If nothing is done, the profession will collapse and the benefits of regulation will not be realized" (Nova Scotia Department of Health and Wellness, 2011, 10). The report made several recommendations, including the credentialing of midwives as a means of obtaining privileges consistent with their scope of practice; the hiring of an experienced midwifery leader as provincial head of midwifery; the provision of funds for "second attendants" to facilitate midwives attending more home births; the consideration of university training for midwives in Nova Scotia; and the establishment of a long-term goal of 20 FTE funded midwifery positions by 2017. Five months later, the government articulated support for the midwifery program and endorsed the report's suggestions to hire a midwifery practice specialist, create a second-attendant program to support midwives, and increase the complement of midwives at the IWK by two full-time equivalent positions. In September 2013 the midwifery program was reinstated at the IWK. Despite the seemingly quick response to the report's recommendations, however, much of the progress made did not result in substantial change. As of July 2015 there are only a handful of second attendants working in Nova Scotia from the IWK site, and the midwifery specialist role in government did not produce the outcomes hoped for by many.

Nova Scotia continues to struggle with the implementation and integration of midwifery.

5.4.4 Medical laboratory technologists

Medical laboratory technology is another field with staffing concerns. A report published in 2001 stated that "Nova Scotia is in the most precarious position of all the provinces ... Urgent action is required to avert a serious shortage in the province" (Canadian Society for Medical Laboratory Science, 2001, 8). The report also underscored the point that while Nova Scotia had the largest percentage of medical laboratory technologists eligible for retirement, it did not have any training programs in the province to produce new ones. By 2015, the province offered a three-year (formerly two-year) diploma program at Nova Scotia Community College, as well as a two-year post-diploma bachelor of health sciences at Dalhousie University. Nonetheless, medical laboratory technologists remain on the list of professions that require "close monitoring" due to potential shortages as retirements continue to mount (37 per cent of the province's 851 medical laboratory technologists in 2015 were over age 50).

5.4.5 Clinical assistants

Unlike some provinces, Nova Scotia does not license physician assistants (also known as physician extenders). However, international medical graduates who have graduated from an accredited medical school and who have passed a qualifying exam have been employed by the QEII Health Sciences Centre since 1995 as clinical assistants. These individuals act in the capacity of residents under the supervision and direction of a department head.

5.4.6 Home care workers

As noted in chapter 1, Nova Scotia has one of the oldest populations and the highest prevalence of chronic disease in Canada. It also is characterized by notably high rates of dementia and disability. At the same time, the province, like other jurisdictions, is attempting to reduce hospital stays in an attempt to control health care spending. This strategy involves increasing the number of long-term-care beds and facilitating seniors' ability to stay at home as long as possible. But, as chapter 4 noted, waiting lists for long-term-care beds are still lengthy; and of those receiving home-care services, 20 per cent had a caregiver in distress (Health Association of Nova Scotia, 2014, 17). The staffing of home-care services is thus a considerable challenge. The 2014 report issued by the Health Association of Nova Scotia clearly outlined the problems underlying the supply of home care workers.

The first issue is the lack of good data regarding the supply of home-care workers. In Nova Scotia, those providing publicly funded home care are required to hold continuing care assistant (CCA) certification. Yet while statistics are kept on the number of individuals graduating from a CCA program in Nova Scotia, the province does not know how many remain in the province, how many of those are employed, and when and how they are employed. While the DHW did support the creation of a registry for CCAs, registration is optional, and uptake has been quite low. Two potential changes to the method of collecting information on the CCA workforce could be to make registration on the CCA registry mandatory, or to conduct a province-wide survey to establish a database on the number and distribution of CCA workers. Another issue is that CCA workers may not be necessary for all forms of home care. Currently, publicly funded home care in Nova Scotia includes personal care, respite care, housekeeping, and meal preparation. Yet these services do not necessarily cover all the tasks that may be required to enable individuals to remain at home: services such as shopping, laundry, banking, driving or accompanying clients to appointments, yard maintenance, and minor home repairs are not covered by provincial home-care services. These services, along with housekeeping and meal preparation, could be performed by personal care workers and home support workers, who are not qualified to provide more specialized personal care and who are paid less than the hourly wage received by CCAs.

Enrolment in provincial CCA training programs peaked in 2010–11 and has been noticeably declining since then. The Health Association of Nova Scotia report identifies a number of reasons for this decline. One is the expiration of the federal-provincial Labour Market Agreement, which provided funding to meet local needs and fill skills gaps. Under this agreement, Nova Scotia was able to provide significant bursaries to those entering CCA programs (amounting to either 70 per cent of tuition costs or $4,000, whichever was lowest). However, funding for this program ended in 2013. At the same time, program fees have been increasing. A program had also been established to recognize existing credentials to facilitate access to CCA training (Recognizing Prior

Learning, or RPL), but many barriers to this program exist (in 2005–06, 41 per cent of CCA graduates went through the RPL; this fell to eight per cent in 2013–14). Overall, enrolment in CCA programs has fallen by about 33 per cent from a high point in 2010–11 (Health Association of Nova Scotia, 2014). As enrolment in training programs falls, however, competition for CCAs has grown from the expanding long-term-care sector, which provides more stable and predictable work environments.

5.5   HHR planning in Nova Scotia

The first comprehensive audit of HHR in Nova Scotia, completed in 2003, noted the lack of a planning framework integrating HHR with the broader forces changing the nature of modern health care systems. To this end, the new Model of Care Initiative in Nova Scotia (MOCINS) was launched in 2008. This strategy focused on "optimizing the utilization of the health care workforce to ensure patients have access to the right providers at the right time," and was seen as "critical to overcoming the current and future workforce shortages and improving quality of care" (Nova Scotia Department of Health and Wellness, 2009, 3). MOCINS was implemented in a series of iterative waves, with each phase followed by an evaluative process. The first implementation phase ran from October 2008 to June 2009, and the second from September 2009 to March 2010. The first phase focused on 14 acute-care units; the second expanded into another 29 units; phase three included maternal-child units; and phase four targeted peri-operative services and emergency care. The strategy itself involves five interrelated approaches:

- *Better utilization of heath care professionals:* The aim here was to ensure that health care professionals were working to full scope of practice. For example, the first evaluation report noted a "significant inconsistency between what a licensed practical nurse could do by licensure and what he or she was allowed to do in the employment setting" (Nova Scotia Department of Health and Wellness, 2009, 13);
- *The redesign of work processes* (e.g., the relocation of supplies closer to the point of care);
- *The use of data on patient population health needs to make staffing decisions:* Understanding the specific needs and risk factors of identifiable populations led to a more efficient composition of health care teams. In one case, the way in which work was originally allocated had meant delays in weaning patients from pain pumps, resulting in

an increased length of stay (Nova Scotia Department of Health and Wellness 2009, 16);

- *The use of integrative technology, and especially comprehensive electronic health records* (see chapter 4); and
- *Ongoing training and mentorship* (e.g., in interprofessional education).

The focus of MOCINS was on patient-centred care, but the operational principles on which the initiative was grounded were *the utilization of needs-based HHR planning* and *the development of interprofessional collaboration*. Both principles leveraged provincial capacity. In the first place, Dalhousie University in Halifax became home to a World Health Organization/Pan-American Health Organization Collaborating Centre on Health Workforce Planning and Research in 2008. This permitted Nova Scotia to contribute substantially to the development of evidence, methodology, and implementation strategies for HHR needs-based planning (Nova Scotia has, for example, contributed to needs-based HHR planning at the national level through the development of the Pan-Canadian Health Human Resources Planning Toolkit and a Health Canada-commissioned project, Competency-Based Health Human Resources Planning for Aging Canadians in Long-Term Care). In the second place, Nova Scotia's small size – often a disadvantage in the development of sophisticated new policy directions permitted it to approach the problem of regulating the collaborative framework for self-regulating professionals in a new way because of the close connection between regulatory health care professional groups in the province.

While provinces such as Ontario impose the requirement to collaborate uniformly on all self-regulating professions, Nova Scotia has developed a regulatory approach to collaborative action between the self-regulated professions that simply *facilitates* collaboration rather than *mandating* it. Under the 2012 Regulated Health Professions Network Act (RHPNA), a statutory body made up of members from all self-regulating professions was given the authority itself to improve the regulation of collaborative behaviour among the health professions (e.g., by authorizing binding interprofessional agreements that set out specific scopes of practice to permit more efficient interprofessional care). Thus Nova Scotia's act enables, but does not dictate, interprofessional collaboration: coordination and cooperation between the professions thus depends on voluntary "bottom up" action rather than prescribed "top down" legislation (Lahey & Fierlbeck, 2016).

The RHPNA was built on the work of the Nova Scotia Regulated Health Professions Network, an informal group founded in 2007. Made up of 22 different regulators, the network formed a working group in 2008 to develop a regulatory framework that would support the development of effective interprofessional relations. The working group released a report in 2009, and the timing was propitious, as it coincided not only with the articulation of the concept of collaborative emergency centres, but also with the evolution of the MOCINS. Thus Nova Scotia's HHR planning strategy emerged contemporaneously with a distinctive regulatory framework for interprofessional collaboration.

5.6 Summary

Like other provinces, Nova Scotia has been attempting to transition to a more collaborative health care system that most effectively utilizes each health profession's scope of practice. Despite the favourable ratio of physicians per population compared to other provinces, Nova Scotians still experience serious barriers regarding access to primary health care. The province has designed some innovative new programs that permit some heath care professions (such as pharmacists and paramedics) to play key roles in the primary health care system. However, other professions (such as nurse practitioners and midwives) are arguably underutilized at present. Nova Scotia has increasingly focused on gathering information on each health care profession, and it now has a much clearer comprehension of the current and future HHR needs of the province. More difficult is the attempt better to integrate programs and services across providers and regions. This issue will be examined more closely in chapters 6 and 7.

Chapter Six

Service and Program Provision

Contemporary health care "systems" are actually complex interrelationships between several discrete subsystems including, most notably, primary health care, specialized/acute care, long-term care, mental health care, and public health. The hospital sector accounts for the largest percentage (29.5) of health care expenditure in Canada (CIHI, 2016a). A key issue across Canada is thus how better to integrate these service delivery systems so that lower-cost services provided in nonhospital settings can provide a more appropriate level of care for patients. Some of the most common policy discussions in health service delivery focus on how to ensure that patients have effective access to community-based primary health care, long-term care, and palliative care when needed so that they are not obliged to use hospital services. A related discussion is how to ensure timely access to support services in the community (such as physiotherapy or mental health services) to enable patients to leave a hospital setting in a timely manner.

Notably, much hospital expenditure is clustered around a very small number of high users. In Quebec, for example, the top 1 per cent of patients accounts for 50 per cent of total hospital expenditure (Côté-Sergent, Échevin, & Michaud, 2016); while in Nova Scotia the top 5 per cent accounts for 64 per cent of insured service expenditure (87 per cent of which is due to inpatient hospitalization) (Kephart et al., 2016). Because these high users tend to have several concurrent chronic health conditions (ibid.), there has been considerable focus on providing effective primary health care to prevent, monitor, and contain these conditions before they develop into a state requiring hospitalization.

Primary care services have four key features: first-contact access; long-term person-centred care; comprehensive care for most individuals' health needs; and coordination of specialized care that cannot be provided within a primary care setting (Starfield, Shi, & Macinko, 2005). "Primary health care" incorporates not only the basic health services provided to patients ("primary care") but also the idea of a population-level system that is designed to promote preventive care as well as manage basic or ongoing health conditions (Muldoon, Hogg, & Levitt, 2006). Primary health care is generally seen as a crucial component of any overarching health care system because it provides effective care at a lower cost, improves health through access to appropriate services, and reduces health inequities across populations (Starfield, Shi, & Macinko, 2005; Starfield, 2010).

But primary health care reform in Canada faces a number of structural obstacles. The structure of federalism prevents a thoroughgoing national level of reform (although it can also facilitate greater experimentation in the provision of primary health). The principle of public payment of private medical practice negotiated as Canada adopted public health insurance has reinforced a structural bias towards fee-for-service payment; and the legislation that served as the foundation for public health insurance also established a policy bias towards GP-based primary health care (Hutchison, Abelson, & Lavis, 2001). Nonetheless, after a period of policy stagnation, primary health care did see some transformation with new primary care models introduced in Quebec (family medicine groups), Alberta (primary care networks), and Ontario (community health centres and family health teams, among others); although primary health care across Canada has been stymied by the slow adoption of information technology, clinical information systems, care coordination, the use of interdisciplinary teams, and participation in quality initiatives (Hutchison, 2008).

As in the case of primary health care, the development of better long-term health options is seen as a means of reducing the utilization of higher-cost hospital services. Again, however, there are structural obstacles to the development of a comprehensive and integrative system of long-term care. The funding of health care following the introduction of hospital insurance focused primarily on hospital facilities, given their cost-shared status; long-term care, with a significant nonmedical component, was to a large extent the financial responsibility of provincial governments alone, often under the purview of community services or social services departments. This led to a considerable fragmentation of care delivery, and an inequality in access to services, both across and within provinces (Hirdes, 2001). Institutionally based long-term care services across Canada are often privately funded, and publicly insured medical services can be billed separately from residential care. There is also considerable debate over the role of home-care services: while they tend to be far less costly than long-term-care facilities or hospitals, they also tend to be subsidized by the caregiving provided by (largely female) family members or by very low-wage caregivers with variable standards of care (Coyte & McKeever, 2001; Grant et al., 2004). A similar kind of fragmentation exists within mental health care, which can be funded through departments of health, community services, justice, or education; provided by either hospitals or community-care agencies; and situated in public, private for-profit, or private not-for-profit spheres.

The role of public health in a high-quality health system is even more complex. Public health is "the organized efforts of society to keep people healthy and prevent injury, illness and premature death" (Office of the Chief Public Health Officer of Canada, 2008), and it often focuses on non-medical determinants of health such as poverty, education, housing, and social networks. And while many studies have drawn clear links between poverty and poor health (Yoshikawa, Aber, & Beardslee, 2012; Evans & Cassells, 2013), the impact of public health is often marginalized by both the inherently political nature of these correlations as well as the way in which evidence is used in public health policymaking (Fierlbeck, 2011; Smith, 2013; Fafard, 2015.) In Atlantic Canada, for instance, public health expenditure (as a percentage of total health care spending) is less than half the national average (Ruggieri, 2015, 355). The attempt to reform "the health care system" is thus incredibly complex, not only because Canada's constitutional framework fragments health care into provincial and territorial units, but also because each provincial health care system is in fact an interlocking "system of systems," each containing its own set of administrative, political, and economic tensions and obstacles to change.

6.1 Public health

When Nova Scotia shifted to a regionalized system in the mid-1990s, the provision of key services and programs in the province became bifurcated, with certain services and programs provided both at the provincial level and through the district health authorities. Public health is illustrative of this dichotomy, with the province spending about $16.5 million directly in 2014–15, and the two health authorities contributing another $29.5 million (see Table 6.1). As in most provinces, the reform of public health in Nova Scotia was driven by the SARS epidemic of 2003, which

Table 6.1 Expenditure summary, programs and services, 2014–15 ($ thousands)

Department of Health and Wellness	
Physician services	789,149
Pharmaceutical services	265,757
Insured services	34,984
Emergency health services	125,104
Continuing care	3,154
Home-care services	236,325
Long-term-care program	554,922
Addiction and medical health programs	9,811
Active living	11,100
Primary care programs	15,881
Public health programs	**16,612**
Provincial programs and initiatives*	130,054
Other programs	23,520
NS Provincial Health Authorities**	
Administration	78,905
Operations	277,642
Inpatient services	488,456
Ambulatory care	247,956
Diagnostic and therapeutic services	299,878
Other acute care expenditures	89,238
Addiction services	38,444
Mental health services	135,208
Public health	**29,592**
Primary health care	13,689
Care coordination	31,380

*These include Breast Screening, Canadian Blood Services, Cancer Care Nova Scotia, Cardiovascular Health NS, Diabetes Care, Emergency Care Fund, Health Association NS, Information Technology Initiatives, Insulin Pump Program, Legacy of Life, NS Hearing and Speech, NS Renal Program, Nursing Strategy, Provincial Blood Coordinating Program, Provincial Drug Distribution Program, and the Reproductive Care Program.
**Nova Scotia Health Authority and IWK.
Source: Nova Scotia, Budget 2015–16, Estimates and Supplementary Detail, pp. 14.2 and 14.13.

identified gaps in capacity, confusion over roles and responsibilities, and issues with coordination within and between jurisdictions. In tandem with the development of the Public Health Agency of Canada (PHAC) in 2005 at the federal level, provinces reevaluated the design and capacity of their respective public health systems. Nova Scotia commissioned a public health review that was published in 2006, and a flurry of activity in public health was evident until 2012.

The key organizational issue underlying public health in Nova Scotia during the era of regionalization was the attempt to provide coordinated, high-quality public health services within an increasingly decentralized structure of governance. With health care governance distributed first into four districts and then into nine, concerns were expressed regarding the capacity of very small DHAs to maintain the level of expertise and capacity required by an effective public health system. The minimum population for a public health unit to manifest a critical mass of expertise and capacity was stated by the province to be around 250,000 (Nova Scotia Department of Health and Wellness, 2012b, 6); yet in Nova Scotia, only one DHA (Capital Health) met or exceeded this figure prior to consolidation in 2015. To move towards critical mass, the province introduced a "shared service area" (SSA) model, which attempted "to create regional functionality out of local structures while the legislation, the funding, and the governance structures are all applied at the DHA level" (Nova Scotia Department of Health, 2006b, xiv). Thus, despite political rhetoric espousing the effectiveness of greater decentralization in health care, the smaller of the nine DHAs were quietly grouped into four SSAs for the administration of public health in an attempt to provide a critical level of expertise and capacity (tellingly, Saskatchewan had already experimented with SSAs, but found them too unworkable) (ibid., 28).

The first public health challenge was the fragmentation of health governance that existed across a number of axes. The first form of fragmentation, noted above, was the division of responsibility and leadership across the DHAs. Both the 2006 public health renewal report and the 2011 mid-course review noted the difficulty of finding and retaining public health directors with appropriate qualifications for smaller jurisdictions. The amalgamation of nine DHAs into a single health authority in April 2015 was designed to solve the problem of finding sufficient public health officials across regions, but the newly-configured Nova Scotia Health Authority (NSHA) retained a public health structure that was divided into four regional administrative areas, and when it was established the health authority still experienced difficulty in finding public health directors in two of these administrative units.

A second form of fragmentation had arisen due to the creation of a free-standing Department of Health Promotion and Protection in 2002. A medical doctor elected premier, John Hamm, had a particular interest in health promotion, and Nova Scotia became the only province to bestow on health promotion both a cabinet voice and a dedicated budget. However, following the analysis of Ontario's structural deficiencies in dealing with the 2003 SARS crisis, Nova Scotia determined that the best way to avoid similar administrative confusion would be to consolidate all public health at the provincial level "with a single point of leadership, visibility, and accountability." This was eventually accomplished in 2012 with the merging of both health and health promotion into a single Department of Health and Wellness. Yet the point of establishing a separate health promotion department in the first place had been to ensure that resources for public health would be clearly protected and not diverted to acute-care services with their perpetual funding shortages. In 2006, 1.2 per cent of Nova Scotia's health care budget was dedicated to public health. The 2006 report called for a doubling of this figure, although it also noted that this would fall short of the 5 to 6 per cent of total public health expenditure that might be optimal for a public health system (Nova Scotia Department of Health (2006b, xvii). Using the figures in Table 6.1, one can calculate that the funds earmarked for public health in Nova Scotia's $4-billion 2014–15 health care budget amounted to only 1.13 per cent of total provincial health care expenditure. Fears that merging health promotion and protection into one health department would result in a diminution, rather than doubling, of public health funding, were thus well-founded.

A third form of fragmentation in Nova Scotia's public health system stems from the decision in 1994 to transfer all of the public health inspectors to the Department of Environment. Following this move, another discrete group of health inspectors was transferred to the Department of Agriculture and Fisheries. This resulted in a profound fragmentation of responsibilities and resources across three departments. To the extent that one set of inspectors focuses on the water supply while the other monitors the food supply, the system can function. But, as the mid-course review pointed out, cases of enteric disease may appear "where the source is unclear and needs to be identified in a timely fashion" (Nova Scotia Department of Health and Wellness, 2012b, 5). In such a circumstance the front line of investigation would have no formal responsibilities to the Department of Health, while those with the training and expertise would not initially be involved at all (leading one observer to label the system "an inquiry waiting to happen"). Organizationally, the province has attempted to facilitate coordination through the creation of the Public Health System Leadership Team, although some of those involved have noted that this body is limited to "the superficial stuff" and that key planning involving budgets, staffing, planning, and evaluation occurs elsewhere in the system (ibid., 14).

If the first challenge for public health in Nova Scotia is fragmentation, a second is in health human resource capacity, although on this point there have been many developments over the past decade. In 2006 the public health renewal report noted that "no PhD-level epidemiologists exist anywhere within the Nova Scotia system" (Nova Scotia Department of Health, 2006b, 45). Saskatchewan in 2006, with a very similar population base, employed five. The report also identified a dearth of public health leaders with formal master of public health (MPH) training. By 2015 the province employed four full-time epidemiologists; and Dalhousie University was not only offering a master's program in public health but had also launched a PhD in public health. In response to the H1N1 pandemic in 2009, Nova Scotia negotiated a "good neighbour protocol" (the first of its kind in Canada) with its health care unions, allowing them to move easily and efficiently between various organizations in the event of staff shortages during a public health emergency (Nova Scotia Department of Health, 2010).

A third major challenge for Nova Scotia's public health system is the lack of an adequate public health IT system. This point was stressed not only in the 2006 and 2012 public health renewal reports, but also in reports by the provincial auditor general in 2008 and 2013. Currently, the province utilizes the ANDS system developed by the Public Health Agency of Canada. However, the ANDS system is effectively obsolete; it is no longer supported and it is difficult to find IT personnel who are conversant with the system. The ANDS system contains minimal data fields; it cannot capture and analyse essential information in sufficient detail; and it has limited reporting capabilities (Nova Scotia Office of the Auditor General, 2013, 64–5). Health administration relies heavily on paper forms and files; even in 2013 the Capital District Health Authority was using free software designed for use in developing countries (ibid., 65). Part of the problem rests with the difficulties encountered by the Panorama project supported by Canada Health Infoway. Nova Scotia was highly involved in Panorama during its first 4 years, investing almost $1.3 million in the system; but by 2010 the province felt obliged to walk away from the project (ibid., 66). The province did weather the 2009 H1N1 flu pandemic with only seven deaths, despite the lack of a computerized vaccination-tracking system. However, as the public health renewal midcourse review cautioned,

> H1N1 was not a scenario in which public health needed to detect an outbreak, investigate it, identify causes and their contacts, and implement control measures on a larger scale. Such an emergency would likely expose to a greater degree existing gaps in information systems, diminishing expertise

within DHAs, role clarity challenges, lack of a public health environmental health program, and limitations in existing epidemiologic capacity. (Nova Scotia Department of Health and Wellness, 2012b, 19)

In 2017, the province announced its intention to adopt a modified version of the Panorama system.

6.2 Primary care

As in other provinces, the primary health care system in Nova Scotia was historically based on independent general practitioners. The province, as noted in chapter 5, has a relatively high ratio of physicians per population. As in all provinces, the ratio has increased steadily over the past three decades, rising from 172 per 100,000 in 1986 to 251 per 100,000 in 2015. And yet, as in most provinces, the distribution of GPs tends to be skewed to metropolitan areas, causing difficulty for inhabitants of small towns and rural areas in securing primary care. Over 61 per cent of GPs practise in Halifax, with 44 per cent of the province's population (CMA, 2015). The professional depopulation of rural areas, especially in Cape Breton, is especially troubling. Access to primary health care is a major political issue. In 2016 only 723,000 Nova Scotians over the age of 12 reported that they had access to a regular health provider (Statistics Canada, 2017), leaving approximately 100,000 individuals without regular primary care. In November 2016 the provincial government established a centralized wait list for those actively seeking family doctors, and a year later the list contained 37,339 names (Corfu, 2017). In November 2017 the NSHA posted job listings for 72 full-time family physicians, 10 part-time family doctors, and 14 family-doctor locums (Ray, 2017).

A 2011 report on primary care in the Capital District Health Authority warned that a "fundamental shift" in the functioning of primary care was crucial to the sustainability of the system; and that "if demand for health services continues at the same rate as today, we can expect to see a 50% increase in patient demand by 2026" (Capital District Health Authority 2011, 3). To meet this demand for primary care, the province has seen the establishment of 35 walk-in clinics, 24 of which are located within the Halifax Regional Municipality alone. Yet the Department of Health and Wellness wants to move away from walk-in clinics and towards a medical-home model of health care. In December 2015, to encourage the growth of collaborative care clinics, the Department of Health and Wellness announced that new doctors to the province would not be allowed to work in walk-in clinics (Colbert, 2015). This led to an outcry by both doctors and the general public, as walk-in clinics were seen as an important stopgap measure to provide immediate primary health care while collaborative care clinics were slowly being established. The number of collaborative care clinics in the province increased significantly between 2008 and 2011, many in rural areas (largely because of incentives to physicians negotiated in the 2008 Physician Master Agreement); but by 2011, the rate of increase in collaborative practices had plateaued. The 2015 Physician Master Agreement was negotiated within an environment of rigid public-service wage increases (see chapter 7), and there was at this point less scope to develop the same kind of incentive structures that were evident in the 2008 document. The move towards a comprehensive primary health care strategy was also delayed because of the transition to a single health authority in 2015, and the reconstitution of the Department of Health and Wellness in 2016. Primary care in 2015 was ceded to the NSHA, which now has the responsibility to draft a provincial primary health care plan.

6.3 Acute care

Nova Scotia has 43 acute-care facilities, and there is a great deal of diversity in size and functional capacity among them. All hospitals offer some degree of emergency care, although this may in some units be provided in the first instance by nurses and paramedics. Some smaller units experience occasional ad hoc closing of emergency services due to staffing shortages (see chapter 4). The most common acute care services, such as cancer surgery, hip and knee replacements, and cataract surgery, are available at hospitals in each of the province's four health care zones, although wait times for these services vary considerably between the four zones. For cataract surgery, for example, the wait time for a consultation in the period from 2015 June 1 to 2015 August 31 was 61 days in Truro and 237 days in Halifax; wait times for surgery following consultation over the same period ranged from 127 days in New Glasgow to 275 days in Bridgewater (Nova Scotia, 2015a). However, some acute care services, such as advanced cardiac care, most internal medicine referrals and interventions, and quaternary care are only available at the Queen Elizabeth II Health Sciences Centre in Halifax.

Compared to other provinces, Nova Scotia had the longest wait times in 2014 for three of the nationally benchmarked procedures (hip replacements, knee replacements, and radiation therapy) and among

Table 6.2 Success in meeting wait times for selected treatments, 2014*

	BC	Alberta	Sask	Man	Ont	Que	NB	NS	PEI	Nfld	Canada
Hip replacement	67%	87%	93%	71%	88%	84%	74%	**58%**	87%	96%	83%
Knee replacement	57%	81%	89%	71%	86%	81%	56%	**44%**	78%	92%	79%
Cataract	70%	71%	88%	63%	81%	88%	89%	**76%**	51%	96%	80%
Radiation therapy	95%	97%	97%	100%	99%	99%	97%	**88%**	90%	98%	98%

*All entries measured against established benchmark of 90%
Source: waittimes.cihi.ca

the longest for the fourth (cataract surgery). For hip replacement, four of 10 provinces either met/exceeded the target of 90 per cent of patients being treated within 182 days, or were within 5 per cent of that target. The national average was 83 per cent; Nova Scotia's average was 58 per cent. For knee replacement over the same period, the national average was 79 per cent; Nova Scotia's average was 44 per cent (see Table 6.2).

The higher demand for these services is largely rooted in the specific demographic challenges that Nova Scotia faces. However, there are also organizational issues underlying these figures. A Patient Access Registry System (PAR-NS) was implemented in 2010 to facilitate a prioritized, province-wide elective surgery waitlist (see chapter 4, section 5.2). An audit conducted by the Auditor General's Office in 2014, however, found that this system was "not consistently used" (Nova Scotia Office of the Auditor General, 2014c, 53). The report also found that available operating room times were not optimally used; that DHAs had not set "realistic organizational performance targets for elective surgery wait times"; that there was no routine reporting of wait times, which meant that there was no regular review to "identify and analyze wait time issues and trends"; that surgeons' offices were "often late in submitting booking formation to hospitals"; and that operating-room policies and guidelines "have not been updated since 2005" (ibid., 54, 59, 50, 64). But the problems were not simply at the DHA level; the report also noted that there was no overall provincial approach to wait-times management and that a common provincial approach was still in the planning stages. Provincially, Nova Scotia established three committees in 2012 to address this issue: the Provincial Perioperative Advisory Committee, which focuses on elective surgery wait times; the Provincial Orthopaedic Working Group, which was established to develop a five-year plan to improve the quality of orthopaedic services; and the Provincial Clinical Services Planning Steering Committee, whose mandate is to coordinate clinical services planning. Nonetheless, in December 2014, the auditor general was quite critical that the province had accomplished little in terms of a systematic provincial approach: "Health and Wellness has no interim targets, no plans, and no defined timeframe by which they plan to reach a one-year maximum wait. There are also no overall Provincial expectations for the district health authority with regards to elective surgery performance" (ibid., 58).

That wait-time management was a political issue was partly due to the Liberals' campaign promise during the 2013 election to reduce wait times for knee and hip replacement surgeries so that they would meet or fall below the national average. After several years in office, the figures for both hip and knee replacements remained relatively constant. Complicating the picture even further, given the administration's commitment not to increase public spending, the Auditor General's Office used the Department of Health and Wellness's own figures estimating that it would take $35 million to move towards the 90 per cent benchmark for hip and knee replacements alone (Nova Scotia Office of the Auditor General, 2014c, 56). In response, the deputy minister of health stated in February 2015 that the province's consolidation of its DHAs would facilitate a more efficient system of surgical treatment (by, for example, more easily using excess operating-room capacity in some of the regional hospitals): "Foundationally, it's a one-Nova Scotia, consolidated, unified health authority that allows us to manage care across artificial boundaries" (Nova Scotia Hansard, 2015a). The deputy minister also noted that the consolidation of the Emergency Health Services (EHS) 20 years previously had led to the establishment of an ambulance service "internationally rated as one of the top 10 in North America" (ibid.).

Despite the province's struggles to address the challenges it faced in acute care, or perhaps because of them, Nova Scotia's emergency health services system has produced a number of innovative features that have been studied and duplicated both nationally and internationally. Prior to 1995, the emergency-response system in Nova Scotia was supplied by private community-based providers (though subsidized by the Department of Health). Of the 54 ambulance operations, many were loss leaders for local funeral homes, and it was not uncommon for hearses or mortuary vans to be used as ambulances. Vehicles, equipment, and supplies were not standardized, and care was provided within a "level of efforts" system without any performance standards. Most paramedics had basic (P1) qualifications and received minimum wage (Nova Scotia Hansard, 2002). This changed dramatically by the mid-1990s. In 1993 a report was commissioned (and presented in April 1994) detailing the inadequacy of service, equipment, and training within the emergency health services system. This led to the creation of the EHS branch within the Department of Health, which consolidated the community-based operations by purchasing the private ambulance operations and replacing the ambulance fleet. The new operator, Emergency Medical Care Inc. (EMC), became the first Canadian ambulance service to be accredited by an international accreditation agency. Nova Scotia also created a single, province-wide communications and dispatch centre (also one of the first in Canada to become accredited) and established an air medical transport (medevac) system. Other supporting programs, such as paramedic training and certification, a trauma program, and a first-responder program were introduced between 1996 and 2000. Within six years, emergency health service delivery in Nova Scotia "evolved from an uncoordinated, fragmented system with uneven service and medical quality to a state-of-the-art, high performance system" (Nova Scotia Office of the Auditor General, 2000, 149). Emergency medicine in Nova Scotia, then, is a unique system, using a failsafe franchise model, a performance-based contract with oversight, province-wide ambulance dispatch, and an integrated air-ambulance component.

The reason for this dramatic change can be traced to the appointment of Dr Ron Stewart as minister of health in 1993. Stewart, a graduate of Dalhousie's Medical School, accepted a residency in emergency medicine in California, and later became head of emergency medicine at the University of Pittsburgh, as well as medical director of Pittsburgh's paramedic system. Returning to Dalhousie in 1989, he was elected to the Legislature in 1993 along with a fellow physician, Dr John Savage, as premier. The development of the system did not come cheaply, nor was it without controversy. EMC, a for-private company owned by the not-for-profit company Maritime Medical Care Inc., was selected to run the day-to-day emergency services operations for the province, which itself does not provide emergency health services directly. EMC was selected without a competitive bidding process, despite an out-of-province company expressing interest because, according to the Department of Health, "the Department lacked financial and operational data upon which to base a request" (Nova Scotia Office of the Auditor General, 2000, 142). As the auditor general noted in his 2000 report,

> There does not appear to be a written evaluation of EMC as a suitable candidate for a Province-wide ground ambulance operator against predetermined evaluation criteria notwithstanding that EMC was a new company

and neither EMC nor the parent company (MMC) had any previous experience in the ambulance business. There also does not appear to have been an analysis of the costs and benefits associated with alternative service delivery by a non-profit or government agency. (ibid., 139)

The cost increases of the new EHS were also significant: from $13.6 million in 1994–5, program costs increased to $53.3 million in 1999–2000 and $125.1 million in 2015–16. The cost drivers were linked to the standardization and overall improvement of common standards and, while a 2001 consultants' report (the Fitch report) accepted that the new service provided good value for money, the auditor general reported in 2007 that the province was lax in monitoring the company's performance and expenditure of public funds (e.g., the province assumed most of the financial risk for the private company operating the service) (Nova Scotia Office of the Auditor General, 2007, 44).

The second wave of emergency-service reform began in 2010. This was driven by two related variables: the first was the underutilization of paramedic services in certain rural areas, and the second was the heavy demand for paramedic services in urban areas. The Long and Brier Island project, for example, began in 2002 because of the low demand for paramedics' services (one emergency call every 2.8 days). Because of the difficulty for this area in providing basic primary care, a pilot project trained paramedics to perform basic primary care services (such as glucose or blood-pressure checks). This was the impetus for the broader utilization of paramedic services in the province, including collaborative emergency centres, the Extended Care Paramedic program in nursing homes, and the use of paramedics in palliative care (see chapter 5). Nova Scotia also became the first province to permit advanced-care paramedics throughout the province to administer thrombolytic drugs to heart attack victims.

The urban problem was based on the poor ambulance turnaround time in emergency departments at the two large hospitals' emergency departments. The benchmark time for paramedics to discharge a patient at an emergency department is 20 minutes or less, 90 per cent of the time. This target was met at the smaller regional hospitals, but in Halifax and Dartmouth this had fallen by 2006 to 20 minutes less than 10 per cent of the time (Nova Scotia Office of the Auditor General, 2007, 54). Because of emergency overcrowding, paramedics were required to remain with their patients at the emergency department, effectively taking them out of circulation for long periods of time. This led the Minister of Health

Maureen MacDonald to commission a report on emergency care restructuring. The report, written by emergency physician John Ross, was the basis for the government report *Better Care Sooner* and included more innovative developments (Nova Scotia Department of Health and Wellness, 2010). Among these was the implementation of standards for emergency departments, making Nova Scotia the first province in Canada to do so. A rapid-assessment unit was put into place in Halifax's main emergency department to divert the treatment of minor cases away from those requiring more serious care. A similar system was then put into place in the Dartmouth emergency department, and the results have been noteworthy: in 2012, only 12 per cent of low-acuity patients saw a doctor within 90 minutes; a year later, after a rapid-assessment system was implemented, this figure rose to 50 per cent (Capital District Health Authority, 2014d). Thus the reform of Nova Scotia's emergency medical care system over 20 years has been a narrative of remarkable progress. At the same time, however, wait times at emergency departments remain an ongoing concern, and progress has been stymied in part due to a poorly developed system of long-term care.

6.4 Long-term care

The components of Nova Scotia's long-term care system include nursing homes/residential care, home care, self-managed care, rehabilitation care, and caregiver-respite programs. The first of these is the most substantial program, with an annual budget of $566 million in 2015–16. Nursing homes provide care for those who are medically stable but who have needs that cannot be met through home care. Residential care is designed for those requiring less intensive care and who have the ability to self-evacuate in the event of an emergency. Nursing homes and residential care facilities in Nova Scotia are privately run, and patients are subsidized by the province on the basis of need. Despite the introduction of new beds, the number of people on the waiting list for admission to these programs in 2017 continues to range from 2,000 to 2,500. To be placed on to the list, individuals must meet with a care coordinator who administers a functional assessment to determine type and level of care, and applicants must have a medical status report completed by their doctor. Those who cannot pay the standard accommodation charge for long-term care must also undergo a financial assessment. The average cost of residential care in 2017 is $250 per diem; the daily rate charged to individuals for "accommodation costs" is between $64.25

and $107.75, depending on the level of care provided. The separation of medical costs (for those requiring medical treatment) and accommodation costs is important, as the provisions of the Canada Health Act stipulate that individuals cannot be charged for "medically-necessary" treatment. Those in long-term care are not expected to pay more than 85 per cent of their assessed income towards accommodation costs (with a minimum retained income of $3,126 per year). If one's spouse remains in the community when one enters a long-term care facility, the spouse retains 60 per cent of the joint family income (minimum of $20,500 per year) as well as maintaining control over all assets. Unsubsidized private care facilities are also available, and costs range from $1,900 to $6,000 per month. In addition to the increasing number of individuals using long-term care facilities, the average length of stay in these facilities has also increased, from 2.2 years in 2006–7 to 2.9 years in 2014–15.

To address the issues of sustainability in the long term care system, the province is, like other jurisdictions in Canada, increasingly focusing on a "home first" strategy. Home care in Nova Scotia is run under the auspices of the Continuing Care branch of the DHW. To access these services, a care coordinator will assess the services for which individuals are eligible based both on need, and on what care a family is able to provide. Approximately 20 per cent of home-care users pay some fee for these services, based both on income and household size. Maximum weekly hours for home care are three for housekeeping, four and a half for personal care, and two for meal preparation. These services amounted to $2.7 million in 2013–14, an increase of 38 per cent over 2006–7, for a total cost of approximately $200 million annually. In 2014–15, $131 million was spent on home-support services, while home nursing amounted to $54 million. More than 22,000 individuals receive home-support services (including nursing care) annually, with approximately 12,000 receiving services on any given day. Moreover, the number of individuals receiving home care who have very high needs has increased by 29 per cent between 2006–7 and 2013–14. The average length of time between the initial home-care referral and service delivery is approximately 56 days, and an average of 398 individuals each month are waiting for home-support services to begin (Nova Scotia, 2015b).

The provision of home care, however, has proven to be highly controversial. The Auditor General's Office has audited Nova Scotia's home-care program three times (1996, 2002, and 2008) and has become increasingly critical of, and frustrated with, the province's lack of response on issues that it has highlighted. Chief among these was the dearth of performance measures and service agreements for the home-care program. The DHW purchases services from more than 20 different organizations: nursing services are almost always provided by the Victorian Order of Nurses (VON), while nonmedical services are generally provided by continuing care assistants (CCAs). In February of 2014, 420 home support workers went on strike in a dispute over wages and were legislated back to work under essential-services legislation the following month. In April 2015, the province attempted to implement a process of competitive bidding for home-care services, which had historically simply been renewed by the DHW, as the auditor general had noted, without performance agreements or a comprehensive system of monitoring. Home-support workers, having been highly mobilized on wage issues, quickly organized a campaign against "for-profit" home care. They argued that tendering contracts would result in large multinational service providers underbidding local firms (potentially using nonunionized workers with few benefits) and providing "assembly-line" care. By the summer of 2015, in the face of public concern, and no doubt to the frustration of the Auditor General's Office, the DHW quietly put its plan to tender home-care services on hold. While the VON announced in November 2015 that it was closing operations in six provinces (including New Brunswick, Prince Edward Island, and Newfoundland and Labrador), Nova Scotia's VON units were not affected.

The province's home-care strategy has other elements as well. The Self-Managed Care Program directly funds adult Nova Scotians with physical disabilities so that they can engage home support and personal care directly. This program is designed so that these individuals can take more control over their lives (although they can also delegate these responsibilities to a third party if they chose). Given that Self-Managed Care clients can receive about 205 hours of care based on a maximum monthly allocation of $3,855.89, compared to home-care clients' monthly maximum of $6,931.50 for 150 hours of home care, it is also a much less expensive program (Nova Scotia, 2015b). In addition, the province provides community-based rehabilitation services through its continuing care strategy. Services include both occupational therapy and physiotherapy, and the clients for whom these services are designed include "those at risk of admission to acute-care facilities, those seeking discharge from such facilities, those with medical or mobility issues who are unable to access public or private outpatient services, and those appropriately seen in the community to address their goals" (ibid., 11). Respite care (either scheduled or on emergency-only basis) is also available, as is adult group day care. Finally, the Supportive Care Program provides additional direct funding for seniors with significant cognitive impairments that interfere with their daily functioning. In this program, home-support services are purchased directly by a client's substitute decision maker, who assumes responsibility for managing the funds and purchasing the services.

6.5 Prescription drugs

As noted in chapter 2 (section 4.3), Nova Scotia offers pharmacare coverage to seniors without private coverage, those receiving income assistance, and those needing treatment for specific diseases (such as cancer, cystic fibrosis, diabetes insipidus, and multiple sclerosis). The province also runs the Provincial Drug Distribution Program, which procures pharmaceuticals from national vendors and distributes them to health care facilities throughout the province. The auditor general notes that drugs purchased through this method are 14.8 per cent less expensive than the prices paid to pharmacies through Nova Scotia's pharmacare programs (Nova Scotia Office of the Auditor General, 2004). In January 2002 the Atlantic Common Drug Review (ACDR) process was established to ensure the quality and effectiveness of pharmaceutical products used by the province. A joint collaboration of the four Atlantic provinces, the ACDR depended on the advice of an expert committee (the Atlantic Expert Advisory Committee) that made listing recommendations for each of the participating provinces. This process was largely, though not entirely, superseded in September 2003 by the National Common Drug Review process (and, in 2010, by the pan-Canadian Oncology Drug Review [pCODR] for drugs used in cancer treatments).

Nova Scotia was the first province to develop a province-wide academic detailing program. The Drug Evaluation Alliance of Nova Scotia (DEANS) has, since 2001, overseen an academic detailing program for physicians. "Academic detailing" is a university-based outreach program in which information is presented to general practitioners by academic medical and pharmacy specialists who research and collate a thorough body of information on specific topics. These topics have, in recent years, included diabetes, COPD, opioids, hypertension, antibiotics, gout, anticoagulants, and contraception. The Nova Scotia detailing program "encourages a culture of critical thinking by informing them of uncertainties and controversies in the interpretation of evidence" (Jin et al., 2012). It is administered by Dalhousie University's Continuing Medical Education programs and is funded by the DHW.

Nova Scotia also runs a drug monitoring program for controlled drugs. The Nova Scotia Prescription Monitoring Program (NSPMP) was established in 1992 as a paper-based program and began to transfer into a secure online system (the Drug Information System, or DIS) in 2013. The program was given a legislative framework in 2005 and, while funded by the DHW, is administered by Medavie Blue Cross. The drugs covered by this program include opioids, barbiturates, psychostimu-lants, cannabinoids, and steroids, although (unlike the prescription monitoring programs in Alberta, British Columbia, and Saskatchewan) benzodiazepines are not included. One function of the NSPMP is to alert pharmacists in real time if an individual requesting a prescription has had another such prescription written by another prescriber and filled within 30 days. This system has "virtually eliminated" the practice of double-doctoring for controlled drugs in Nova Scotia (Furlan et al., 2014). The DIS will also alert a pharmacist if a prescription is related to stolen prescription pads. Another function is to identify individuals who have received prescriptions from three or more prescribers; these reports are generated retrospectively and are sent to prescribers. Infor-mation produced by the NSPMP can be requested by law enforcement agencies. The NSPMP processes between 350 and 500 requests each year from law enforcement agencies regarding information pertaining to criminal investigations (Bradley, 2016). Finally, the NSPMP generates a report every 56 days on prescribers who have exceeded a particular prescribing threshold on monitored drugs. Prescribers can also request data to compare their prescribing patterns to provincial and regional averages. Prescribers who generate prescriptions for monitored drugs above an undisclosed threshold are identified and are referred to the Practice Review Committee of the Prescription Monitoring Board, which provides peer review of flagged prescribing practices. The Prac-tice Review Committee may also refer prescribers to their appropriate regulatory college.

Outcomes for the NSPMP have been mixed. On the one hand, doc-tors referred to the College of Physicians and Surgeons have generally subsequently modified their prescribing practices, "suggesting this was a deterrent to inappropriate prescribing" (Nova Scotia Office of the Audi-tor General, 2012b). The College of Physicians and Surgeons has also permanently banned physicians who do not respond to practice reviews from prescribing controlled drugs. On the other hand, the program relies heavily on manual review, which means that staff are frequently overwhelmed by the data provided by the computerized system (ibid.). In February 2016 one doctor was arrested after it was determined that she prescribed 50,000 Oxyneo and oxycodone pills which she picked up directly from pharmacists, stating that it was on behalf of her patients. An external audit found that, while the Prescription Monitoring Program had flagged this behavior for some time, the monitoring program's medical consultant had kept his notes on the case private, so no official intervention was made for six years (Chiu, 2016).

6.6 Workers' Compensation Board programs

The Workers' Compensation Board of Nova Scotia, established in 1917, currently insures 325,000 workers and provides insurance for 18,700 employees. Compared to other provinces, Nova Scotia has among the highest injury rates and the longest periods of time off work. The highest rates of injury in the province occur in the home care and long-term care sector. Overall, the province pays out on approximately 50,000 claims per year (Workers' Compensation Board of Nova Scotia, 2015). The health care benefits offered by the Workers' Compensation Board in Nova Scotia include hospital care; physician, physiotherapy, and chiropractor visits; surgery; prescription drugs; dental expenses; travel-for-care expenses; and items such as braces or crutches. It also covers earning replacement benefits, return-to-work plans, and survivor benefits. Because workplace disability can be a result of long-term exposure to various factors, the insurance offered by the Workers' Compensation Board in Nova Scotia provides a number of exceptions to the requirement of establishing proof of causality when making a claim. One example is the principle of "presumptive benefits" for firefighters that was introduced in 2003. As epidemiological studies demonstrate a statistically significant increase in the rate of certain cancers for firefighters, individual firefighters do not have to prove a connection between their illness and their workplace for these cancers. Between 2003 and 2014, 60 presumptive cancer benefits were approved (Nova Scotia Hansard, 2014). Similarly, coal miners in Nova Scotia enjoy the principle of "automatic assumption" where it is automatically assumed that any individual working in a coal mine (or in similar conditions) for 20 or more years and who experiences permanent impairment or loss of lung function has this illness due to workplace conditions. A more recent policy change has been the way in which "psychological injury" has been interpreted. Following changes to the *Diagnostic and Statistical Manual of Mental Disorders* (fifth edition) in 2013 regarding post-traumatic injury, which now distinguishes between acute onset and cumulative onset, emergency workers can now submit claims for situations in which multiple events, though traumatic, did not result in an immediate acute reaction but did have a cumulative effect resulting in a final acute event.

6.7 Mental health care

More so than any other area of health service provision, mental health care services have been fragmented due to issues of jurisdiction both vertically and horizontally. The vertical fragmentation is both regional and federal, and can be traced back to the vestiges of the British Poor Laws incorporated by Nova Scotia's colonial governors. The province's first mental hospital was opened in 1858, and by 1875 Mount Hope Hospital housed more than 300 patients, many of whom came from municipalities across the province. These municipalities were responsible financially to the hospital for the upkeep of these patients, although the hospital was rarely able to secure these funds: in 1884, one commissioner wrote that "[a] very urging letter was sent to each municipality last year, but as the receipts show, without any appreciable effect" (quoted in Leighton, 1982, 25).

By 1890, 11 mental hospitals had opened in municipalities throughout the province. By 1904 the number had expanded to 17 (Torrey & Miller, 2007), and municipalities were once again held responsible for providing mental health services. But this shifted dramatically after 1948, when the federal government (under the direction of Health Minister Paul Martin, Sr) established federal health grants that, among other things, were directed to assessing mental health needs, training health care personnel, building infrastructure, and developing research capacity. In exchange, however, provinces were directed to admit patients to these hospitals free of charge (Fingard & Rutherford, 2005). But few municipalities had the capacity to underwrite the total cost of these institutions, and the province stepped in to cover a third of municipal mental hospitals' costs. The 1957 Hospital Insurance and Diagnostic Services Act did not, however, cover mental hospitals, and the province found it difficult to support 17 separate institutions. By 1966, the province closed or amalgamated the municipal mental hospitals so that only four fully funded hospitals remained. This coincided with the trend to deinstitutionalization, which was partly driven by philosophical shifts in the discipline, but was also due to adjustments in funding patterns.

In 1975 New Brunswick negotiated an arrangement with Ottawa in which mental patients requiring long-term rehabilitation and treated in the community were eligible for funding under the Canada Assistance

Plan (Fingard & Rutherford, 2005, 2011). Nova Scotia soon seized on this funding source as well, and the number of individuals treated in psychiatric hospitals fully funded by the province continued to decrease. Yet this move underscored the growing horizontal fragmentation of mental health care across an increasing number of government departments at the provincial level. Historically, mental health generally involved (in addition to the Department of Health) the Department of Social Services (now Community Services), as well as the provincial attorney general's office, for cases involving dangerously violent or criminal behaviour (ibid.). Currently, with mental health programs for youth focused increasingly on placing mental health programs and professionals in the schools (such as the SchoolsPlus program), with an increased emphasis on housing as a key component of long-term addiction rehabilitation, and with initiatives such as the Mental Health Court Program, mental health care is dependent on a high degree of collaborative involvement by the DHW, Community Services, Justice, and Education.

Until the merger of health authorities in 2015, each DHA was responsible for developing and running its own mental health programs and services, although certain services (such as the early identification and intervention programs for children with autism) were fairly consistent across the province. In general, each DHA offered some form of group therapy, family therapy, inpatient care, community-based assisted living services, crisis response, senior mental health services, mental health assessment for adults, children, and youth, and senior outreach, although the particular articulation of each varied across districts (Nova Scotia, 2011). However, eligibility for these services, and points of access to these services, varied from DHA to DHA. As service provision was transferred to a single provincial health authority in 2015 (with additional services at the IWK), an important issue was how to retain services targeted to distinctly local needs. Interestingly, Nova Scotia is the only province in Canada with mental health standards although, as the Auditor General's Office noted, the province has not dedicated sufficient funding, nor provided adequate monitoring, to give these standards real substance (Nova Scotia Office of the Auditor General, 2010a). Currently, the province spends approximately 3.4 per cent of its health budget on mental health care (ibid., 50). In 2012, an advisory committee on mental health and addictions strategy noted lengthy wait times for those attempting to access mental health services, as well as difficulties for those navigating assessment, treatment, and care once in the system (Nova Scotia, 2012b). In response, the province introduced the Choice and Partnership Approach, which is based on problem-solving and offering choices to patients.

6.8 Dental health care

Nova Scotia has had a Children's Dental Plan since 1974. Renamed the Children's Oral Health Program (COHP) in 1997, the program was amended in 2002 to make the COHP the insurer of last resort. While the eligible age range itself shifts a great deal, the COHP covers all children in the eligible age range, but only if they do not have private insurance coverage. The program will also cover any shortfall if private insurance does not cover the full amount. The Oral Health Advisory Group noted that "there does not seem to be a program in any jurisdiction that is structured like Nova Scotia's COHP" (Nova Scotia Department of Health and Wellness 2015b, 9).

The COHP is a dental-office-based program for children under a specified age. It covers one dental examination, two X-rays, fillings, one preventive service (such as cleaning), and nutritional counselling. Extractions are not usually covered. In 2013, the age of eligibility increased to 14 and was scheduled to increase every year until children were covered to the age of 17. However, the Oral Health Advisory Group in 2015 observed that while the costs of the COHP increased significantly, "the percentage of eligible children accessing the COHP remains at less than 50%" (Nova Scotia Department of Health and Wellness, 2015b, 10). The COHP was originally designed to support diagnostic, preventive, and restorative services but, as the Oral Health Advisory Group discovered, 56.5 per cent of the costs of the program are in restorative services, while the remainder are split between preventive and diagnostic services. Were children to utilize more preventive services, the cost of restorative services could be minimized; thus, the advisory group recommended that the focus of the COHP shift from restorative services to prevention (ibid., 13). However, the advisory group recommended shifting the focus to preventive care through "specific additions, deletions, and adjustments to the insured dental procedure codes" rather than through the expansion of dental hygiene within the primary health care system (ibid., 14). There are seven independent dental hygiene practices in Nova Scotia, including three mobile-service practices. However, there is no coverage of dental hygienists' services under existing public dental service plans, even though the Dental Hygienists Act of 2009 removed the stipulation that dental hygienists had to work under the supervision of a dentist (College of Dental Hygienists of Nova Scotia, 2014). In 2015 Nova Scotia had 14.5 FTE positions for dental hygienists working in the Public Health branch, but these were specifically directed towards working on health promotion and community health initiatives. Dalhousie University's school of dentistry provides a number of programs in which services are offered by supervised students. These include half-price services at the dentistry school and outreach programs (including one for the frail elderly and one for refugees at the Halifax Refugee Clinic).

6.9 Targeted services

6.9.1 First Nations

Health data regarding the Nova Scotia Mi'kmaq population has been limited and inconsistent. A 2007 survey found that while Mi'kmaq adults tended to have slightly higher levels of the most common chronic health conditions, the rate of diabetes was generally twice as high as the overall Nova Scotia population (see Figure 6.1). Data released in 2016 showed that rates of diabetes for indigenous people between 20 and 39 years of age were five times higher than the rate for the overall population of Nova Scotia (MacLennan, 2016). This correlates to significantly higher levels of obesity among Nova Scotia Mi'kmaq: according to the 2007 survey on Mi'kmaq health, 50 per cent of female Mi'kmaq and 39.7 per cent of male Mi'kmaq were obese (Mi'kmaq Health Research Group, 2007, 109), compared to the Nova Scotia nonindigenous average of 22.9 per cent and the Canadian nonindigenous average of 16.9 per cent (Public Health Agency of Canada & CIHI, 2011, 9). Of Mi'kmaq in Nova Scotia, 59.1 per cent reported smoking daily (compared to the average Nova Scotia rate of 27 per cent), and 25.2 per cent of Mi'kmaq reported smoking an average of 25 or more cigarettes per day (Mi'kmaq Health Research Group, 2007, 126).

The relationship of First Nations and the government of Nova Scotia regarding the provision of health care has been a very long and complex one. In 1800, a Joint Committee of the Assembly and Council of Nova Scotia was convened to examine the situation of "the Indians in their present distress." After two hundred years of European settlement, by the early 1800s the local Indigenous populations had considerably less access to traditional hunting and fishing areas and increased exposure to waves of disease. Twohig (1991) documents outbreaks of smallpox in 1800–2, cholera in the 1830s, tuberculosis in 1841, infectious hepatitis in 1846–7, diphtheria in 1860, and whooping cough in 1891 among the Mi'kmaq in Nova Scotia. Venereal disease, measles, typhus, rheumatic fever, and alcoholism were also commonly reported in these communities. By 1847, the Indian commissioner described "a discouraged and spirit-broken people," reduced "to the extreme of wretchedness" (ibid., 74). From the early

Figure 6.1 Chronic health conditions, Mi'kmaq and Nova Scotia average

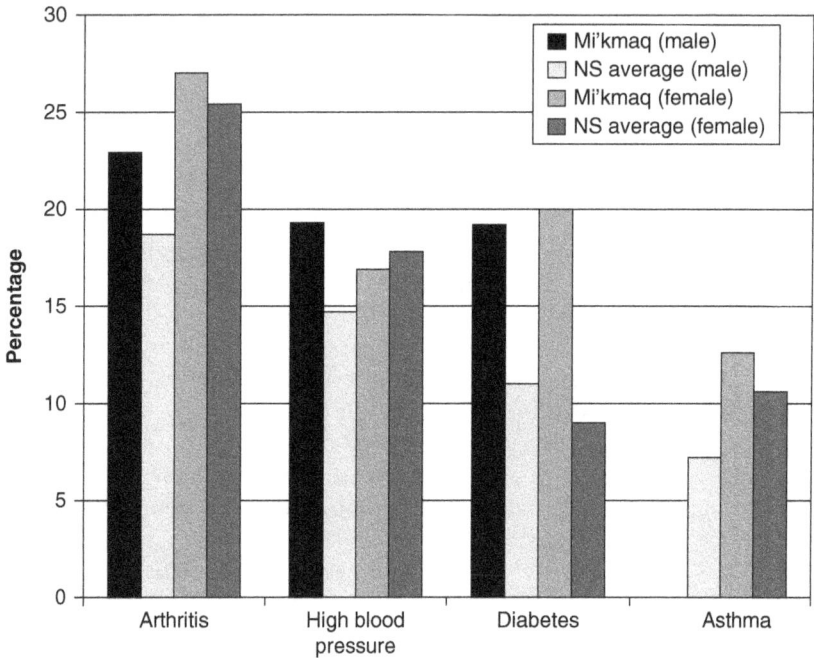

*No data available for asthma for Mi'kmaq males.
Sources: Mi'kmaq Health Research Group, The Health of the Nova Scotia Mi'kmaq
Population (http://www.unsi.ns.ca/wp-content/uploads/2015/07/ns-rhs-report-07.pdf);
Nova Scotia Department of Health and Wellness, Nova Scotia Diabetes Report 2011
(http://diabetescare.nshealth.ca/sites/default/files/files/NSDMReport2011.pdf); Nova Scotia Department of Health, Chronic Conditions in Nova Scotia (http://novascotia.ca/dhw/
publications/annual-statistical-reports/CCHS_Chronic_Conditions.pdf).

1800s until Confederation, the health of First Nations was a matter of
direct colonial responsibility. Health care to the nonmilitary settler population was quite poor during this period, and health services provided to
the indigenous populations were also very limited. What is more remarkable, as Twohig (1996) notes, is that some of the most prominent physicians in the province were involved in providing health services to the
Mi'kmaq population (including Sir Charles Tupper, who would become
the first president of the Canadian Medical Association as well as premier of Nova Scotia and, later, prime minister of Canada). Because this
time period was quite formative for the modern discipline of licensed

medicine, Twohig suggests that the provision of medical care to a very marginalized population was not only due to doctors' traditional sense of "service to the indigent" or to the guaranteed payment of services from the Indian Grant (which was in fact often disputed by the Legislative Assembly), but also a strategy by licensed physicians to advance their profession (against numerous nonlicensed medical practitioners) by establishing formal connections with state authority (ibid., 342).

After Confederation, jurisdiction for First Nations became a federal responsibility. And while health care was not seen as part of formal treaty obligations, the incidence of communicable disease on treaty lands led Ottawa to establish the Medical Services Branch for the Department of Indian Affairs (renamed the First Nations and Inuit Health Branch in 2000). As in other provinces, Indigenous health care is framed by the 1979 Indian Health Policy document, the 1989 Health Transfer Policy, and the 2008 Aboriginal Health Transition Fund (of the $200 million of the fund distributed across Canada over 5 years, Nova Scotia received $3 million). Nationally, these policies have been aimed at improving the health status of First Nations, improving the relationship between First Nations and federal/provincial governments, and increasing the capacity of First Nations to evaluate health needs and to provide health services.

One of the greatest difficulties for Nova Scotia in developing a self-directed indigenous health strategy is the small size and fragmented nature of the Indigenous community. In 2014, the total Indigenous population comprised 2.7 per cent of the province's population. These individuals are distributed across 34 reserve locations comprising 13 Mi'kmaq communities. All but two of these communities have populations of less than 1,500; the smallest has only 283 members. Many of those with formal Indian status live off-reserve. This leads to a number of logistical problems when attempting to design optimal services. For example, the ideal long-term care facilities, according to a survey of indigenous respondents, would be culturally specific and would be located within the individual's community of residence. With only 45 indigenous individuals across Nova Scotia in long-term care, however, the critical mass does not exist to provide these facilities (Nova Scotia, 2010d). Also, as funding for programs is often on a per-capita basis, smaller communities find it particularly difficult to provide a wide range of good services.

In December 2017, Indigenous and Northern Affairs Canada (INAC) was divided into Indigenous Services Canada (ISC) and Crown-Indigenous Relations and Northern Affairs Canada (CIRNAC). The First Nations and Inuit Health Branch (FNIHB) was transferred from Health

Canada to ISC. The FNIHB provides some primary and public health services across Canada (particularly in remote areas), but in Nova Scotia its principal function is to provide Non-Insured Health Benefits (NIHB) to status indigenous populations. These benefits include drugs, dental care, medical supplies, mental health services, vision care, and medical transportation. Primary and hospital care for First Nations members is provided through the provincial health care system (MSI); NIHB are only for health services or goods that are not insured by the province.

There is some cost-sharing between provincial and federal governments. All indigenous individuals are eligible for long-term care under the same criteria applicable to all Nova Scotians (i.e., the province will cover all insured medical costs in long-term care facilities). The Assisted Living Program offered by ISC, however, will also fund the non-medical care component of long-term care for those who are normally resident on-reserve and who have care needs that can no longer be met at home. And, according to Jordan's principle, any government department of first contact will pay for the service for a First Nations child so that care is not compromised by administrative disputes between jurisdictions.

Many of the projects initiated under the aegis of the 2008 Aboriginal Health Transition Fund were specific to particular DHAs. One major initiative, the attempt to integrate continuing care, was completed in 2015. Another initiative that stemmed from the Aboriginal Health Transition Fund is a health awareness project assisting indigenous people living off-reserve to navigate access to health services. This project has been undertaken jointly by the DHW and the Native Council of Nova Scotia. The Health Fund also provided the impetus for the Unamak'i Client Registry Data Sharing Agreement between five Cape Breton bands, the DHW, INAC, Dalhousie University, Medavie Blue Cross, Health Canada and the Public Health Agency of Canada. Work to create the registry began in 2012, and the first results from the registry were reported in 2016. The registry links data from INAC's registry system with data from the province's MSI (health insurance) registry, providing a thorough picture of health data on which to base health programs for Cape Breton's indigenous community Other programs have more recently been developed from other funding sources. One of these is the 2009 Aboriginal Health Sciences Initiative, co-sponsored between Dalhousie University and the Johnson Scholarship Foundation to encourage members of those belonging to indigenous communities in the Maritimes to consider careers in health-related fields. Another is the Transformational Research in Adolescent Mental Health project established in 2014 and funded by the Access Canada Network. Under this initiative, the Eskasoni community in Cape Breton is one of 13 sites across Canada to receive funding for mental health services for 12- to 25-year-olds in the community.

6.9.2 African Nova Scotians

Very little systematic research has been done on the health profile of the African Nova Scotian communities. In 2008 a study using several complementary databases examined specific health indicators for one predominantly Black community (Preston, which is 86.2 per cent African Nova Scotian) and compared it to rural communities with little or no African Nova Scotian populations. The study found rates of circulatory disease, diabetes, and psychiatric disorders that were 13 to 43 per cent higher in the African Nova Scotian community. These rates are consistent with those in the African diaspora in the United States and United Kingdom (Kisely, Terashima, & Langille, 2008). The African Nova Scotian population has deep historical roots in the province and, as a consequence, is largely rural rather than urban. The total African Nova Scotian population is approximately 20,790 (2.1 per cent of the population), of which about 3,205 live in Halifax.

The first Black settlers in Nova Scotia were brought as slaves throughout the eighteenth century, although the Nova Scotia Archives notes that in 1767, 194 free Black persons were living in the colony (Nova Scotia Archives, 2016a). Black settlement to Nova Scotia occurred in four waves. The first was in 1783, subsequent to the American Civil War, when approximately 3,000 Black Loyalists arrived in Nova Scotia when the British promised freedom to the former slaves of rebelling American colonists. White Loyalists also fled to Nova Scotia, bringing their slaves with them. In 1792, a large proportion of the Black Loyalists (around 1,190) emigrated from Nova Scotia to Sierra Leone. Four years later, 600 "Maroons" from Jamaica arrived in Nova Scotia and were offered the lands recently vacated by the Black Loyalists. By 1800, however, many of the Maroons themselves departed for Sierra Leone (ibid.). The third wave of Black settlement was precipitated by the War of 1812, and approximately 2,000 "Black Refugees" settled in Nova Scotia. This group formed the basis of the province's current African Nova Scotian communities, and most of this group settled in small settlements throughout the province (although one remaining record from 1812 notes that almost one-sixth of the population of Halifax at this time was Black [ibid.].)

A final wave of Black immigration occurred in the early 1900s and consisted largely of Caribbean immigrants settling in Cape Breton to work in the steel mills and coal mines. The small rural communities settled historically by Black immigrants were often quite isolated and of poor agricultural quality. The largest urban community, Africville, which grew up on the outskirts of Halifax from the mid-1800s, was in proximity to the city's abattoirs, prison, infectious-diseases hospital, night-soil disposal pits, and open dumps. In the mid-1960s, the land was expropriated and bulldozed, and inhabitants were relocated to public housing areas within the city (Nova Scotia Archives, 2016b).

Some initiatives and supports have been implemented to support the health of African Nova Scotians. In 2002 the Health Association of African Canadians (superseding the Black Women's Health Network) was formed to address the health issues of the African Canadian community in Nova Scotia; and in 2014 the Nova Scotia Brotherhood Initiative, based on a successful program in Chicago, began to establish culturally specific health clinics for African Nova Scotian men. Dalhousie University, in conjunction with the Johnson Scholarship Foundation, has created a program to promote leadership in the health professions for African Nova Scotians. Cancer Care Nova Scotia investigated the experience of African Nova Scotians with cancer in 2001 and followed up with a focus group in 2012. The group reported progress in access to education, information, and resources in their own community; better knowledge of the role of cancer patient navigators; improved cultural competency on the part of health care providers; and a greater sense of empowerment in relation to the health care system. Nonetheless, it also reported that African Nova Scotian health care users experienced systemic racism, encountered delays in accessing service, and faced barriers in respect to transportation and medical costs (Cancer Care Nova Scotia, 2013).

6.9.3 Acadian Nova Scotians

Nearly all francophones living in Nova Scotia are bilingual, and the number of French speakers in the province has been steadily declining. Nonetheless, 77 per cent of French speakers in Nova Scotia hold that government services should be provided in French, and that the linguistic rights of French speakers in the province must be respected (Aubé, 2013, 23). The Fédération acadienne de la Nouvelle-Écosse has also been able to access federal funds to support provincial initiatives, such as the 2002 study of French health care services in Nova Scotia. Despite the fact that Nova Scotia is not formally a bilingual province, the province initiated a French-language service plan for health care, which it continues to update every two years.

The Acadians of Nova Scotia are the descendants of French settlers who arrived in Nova Scotia throughout the seventeenth century and who were largely deported in the middle of the eighteenth century. Throughout the nineteenth century exiles returned to the province and, by the late 1800s, had developed a strong cultural identity that was able to exert political influence on provincial policy throughout the twentieth century. One reflection of this is the establishment of an office of "Acadian Affairs" in the provincial government. There is also a discrete Acadian school board that runs a separate stream of French-only (not immersion for anglophones) education. The Acadian population in Nova Scotia is thus small but politically significant. While the overall French-speaking population in Nova Scotia amounts to 3.7 per cent of the population (around 31,000 individuals), this includes non-Acadian francophones as well as Acadians.

Currently, the DHW provides an online directory of French-speaking primary health care providers. The 811 telephone health service (HealthLink) is available in French, as is the help line of the Gambling Support Network, which launched in March 2015. Three seats in Dalhousie's Medical School are funded specifically for francophone students, as are two pharmacy seats. The province employs 70 bilingual paramedics and is home to six bilingual nursing homes and two bilingual long-term care facilities. Nova Scotia actively recruits francophone medical students from Quebec and offers grants to French-speaking nursing students to encourage them to seek employment within the province. Many documents pertaining to health services are translated into French. The province employs a coordinator for French-language services to liaise between the francophone community and the DHW, and the minister and deputy minister met with this community to "discuss opportunities for French-language services within the new health authority" when the NSHA was established.

6.10 Palliative care

In Nova Scotia, 60 per cent of deaths occur in hospital; only 18 per cent occur at home (Nova Scotia Hospice Palliative Care Association, n.d.). While the province has the largest proportion of the population over age

65, there is no province-wide system of palliative care. Most communities offer some form of palliative care, but there is no consistent minimum standard of care across the province; there is no single point of access into the palliative care system; and there is little quality assurance governing the programs that do exist. Currently, most palliative care is delivered through the existing home-care program and includes both nursing and home support (personal care, respite, and housekeeping). Fees are determined according to income. In 2012, Nova Scotia introduced its Palliative Home Care Medication Coverage Program. Those eligible must be living at home, diagnosed with a life-threatening illness, and assessed as being within 6 months of death. There is no cost to the patient for medications under this program, but for those with private insurance the Palliative Home Care Medication Coverage Program is the payer of last resort. There are 33 palliative-care services across Nova Scotia (some run by the VON), but there are no free-standing residential hospices. However, Hospice Halifax began to develop a residential hospice in Halifax in 2017, with the cost shared between the provincial health authority and the hospice society.

In 2014 the province released *Integrated Palliative Care: Planning for Action in Nova Scotia*. The report's rationale was based on the effective integration of primary, secondary, and tertiary health care with emphasis on the preferences of patients and caregivers. Support for patients and caregivers adapts as each patient's condition advances and changes. The report notes the need to standardize processes, establish a single point of entry, and build capacity and partnerships within the community for hospice care (Nova Scotia, 2014d). Progress has been made since 2014 towards a more comprehensive palliative care strategy in Nova Scotia, including the appointment of a palliative care coordinator. This progress has been expedited by two considerations: first, a residential-hospice bed is less than half the cost of an acute-care bed, while the cost of a home-care bed is even less (Hospice Society of Greater Halifax, 2013). Second, the 2015 centralization of health authorities has simplified the organizational task of standardizing palliative-care practices across the province.

6.11 Assisted reproduction

Fertility treatments are not covered by public health insurance in Nova Scotia. However, the treatments are available on an out-of-pocket basis at the Atlantic Assisted Reproductive Therapies (AART) clinic in Halifax. Established in the 1980s by the Department of Obstetrics and

Gynecology at Dalhousie University, AART provides a comprehensive range of reproductive therapies. Patients can be referred by their GPs or specialists such as gynecologists, but they do not need a referral to access the clinic. All clinic doctors are board-certified physicians with subspecialty training in reproductive endocrinology, and have teaching appointments or research roles at Dalhousie University. AART also offers outreach programs in St. John's and Corner Brook in Newfoundland and Labrador; Charlottetown in Prince Edward Island; and Moncton, Saint John, and Fredericton in New Brunswick.

6.12 Summary

As chapter 7 will describe in more detail, the way in which health care services in Nova Scotia were administered after April 2015 changed quite substantially. Until 2015, most services were designed and provided through one of the nine DHAs, although certain kinds of services (such as cancer care) were administered both at the regional and at the provincial level. The expectation underlying the reforms was that a more centralized planning process and administrative system would be able better to integrate service delivery (e.g., between primary health care and mental health care, or between acute care and long-term care). However, because of the 2015 amalgamation of DHAs, and the complementary reform of the DHW in 2016, the actual redesign of many services themselves was deferred. The strategic planning for many key program areas (including primary health care, long-term care, and mental health care) following these reforms was, at the beginning of 2017, still in development.

The redesign of primary health care is to a large extent the cornerstone for the restructuring of other health care services. The vision is to have a primary health system based on collaborative-care practices. These practices, encompassing a mix of health professionals working effectively in their respective scopes of practice, would serve as permanent medical homes for patients. By taking individuals' long-term wellbeing into account, these practices would focus on preventive as well as curative care, leading ideally to a healthier population and a more cost-effective health care system. Yet administrative reorganization itself is not sufficient to achieve this objective. One key barrier that still exists is the lack of a clear understanding of which groups are responsible for which outcomes. Another major obstacle is the way in which some services (such as nonphysician health professionals working in collaborative care teams, or non-face-to-face GP consultations) are funded. Until these issues are addressed, it is difficult to move forward in the development of collaborative-care-based health care. Uncertainty (e.g., in the scope of practice for GPs relative to other health care professionals and medical specialties or in remuneration for electronic tasks) leads to resistance to change, which in turn sets up obstacles to the development of formal collaborative models. Nova Scotia's engagement in health care restructuring throughout 2015 and 2016 was justified on the grounds that such rationalization was essential in moving towards a more effective model of health care provision. Nonetheless, as chapters 7 and 8 will explain in more detail, moving from a regionalized model of health care administration to one based on a single health authority is simply the beginning, rather than the end, of such a process.

Chapter Seven

Recent Health Reforms

Nova Scotia's health care system underwent very significant reforms in 2015 and 2016. Both were large-scale administrative and organizational reforms addressing the need to coordinate health care planning, integration, and funding across regions and sectors. On April 1, 2015, the province's nine regional health authorities were merged into the Nova Scotia Health Authority (NSHA) (with the IWK Health Centre remaining a discrete administrative entity). For the following year, the Department of Health and Wellness (DHW) experienced significant organizational restructuring to support the new health authority. The scope and scale of these larger reforms have meant that more specific reforms at the program and service level were deferred as the larger projects were completed. Because of this, major programmatic changes in areas such as primary care, mental health care, long-term care, and long-term capital planning were still in the planning stages in 2017.

In their study of health care reforms in Canadian provinces, Lazar, Lavis, Forest, and Church (2013) suggest that successful reforms had certain common elements. First, a general sense of fiscal crisis was a useful prerequisite "to force open the windows of opportunity and allow in the reform winds" (12). Second, major reforms were supported by a sense of democratic legitimacy. Lazar et al. note that such reforms were generally undertaken by first-time governments that had made strong electoral commitments to the reform prior to taking office (179, 184). Third, a majority government was highly advantageous in seeing reforms through to completion (196). Fourth, successful provinces were adept in organizational preparedness and had a systematic plan for achieving their reforms (241, 251). And, finally, the kinds of reform plans undertaken were more "technical" than "political": in other words, they took place at a higher administrative level and did not significantly affect the day-to-day relationship between patients and health care providers (189, 243).

The theoretical analysis presented by Lazar et al. is, for the most part, validated by the major restructuring in health care administration executed by the Liberal government in 2015 and 2016. These administrative reforms will be discussed in more detail in the following sections. In discussing reform, however, it is also useful briefly to note the one significant reform to the delivery of health care services in Nova Scotia that has occurred since 2010: the shift to collaborative emergency centres (CECs) beginning in 2010. The NDP government was elected in 2009 not so much for what it promised to do in health care as for what it promised *not* to do: close down small rural hospitals. This led to the systematic restructuring of emergency services both within rural and urban areas, a process that was much more "political" than "technical" to the extent that it very palpably affected the health care choices of individuals in a very granular manner. While the phenomenon of CECs has not been closely studied from the angle of policy development, it is likely that the success of this reform was due to the incremental development of CEC units across the province, close consultation with communities, and a clear message that *staffing* changes were not *service* changes (and, rather, that staffing changes meant improvements in service). In this case, again following the account of Lazar et al., the appointment of a policy champion (Dr John Ross) "both created and reflected a sense of urgency" that helped to propel and legitimize the reforms (2013, 182).

7.1 The consolidation of district health authorities and the creation of the Nova Scotia Health Authority

As Lazar et al. suggest, any political party with health reform in its sights must make it an explicit issue when running for office. In the 2013 electoral campaign, the provincial Liberal party made few categorical policy promises, but it did commit both to the amalgamation of district health authorities and to a balanced budget (Liberal Party of Nova Scotia, 2013). The two components were not discrete objectives but were closely linked, as the party argued that the consolidation of DHAs would in and of itself lead to cost savings of 13 million dollars (CBC, 2014a). The party did not specify precisely how these cost savings would arise, although it did argue that the DHAs were top heavy with highly paid administrators (Nova Scotia Hansard, 2013). Administrative costs underlying Nova

Scotia's public health care system were actually falling before the Nova Scotia Liberal party was elected (CIHI, 2015c, Table D.3.3.1). Moreover, Nova Scotia, with nine health authorities, spent considerably less overall in administrative costs than Alberta, with a single health authority (ibid., see also Table D.3.9.1). Nonetheless, Nova Scotia still spent a slightly larger proportion of its health care budget on administration than most other jurisdictions (approximately 4 per cent of total health care spending, or about one percentage point higher than many other jurisdictions) (ibid.)

The stance on amalgamation was in stark contrast to the policy recommendations that had been articulated over the previous two decades in Nova Scotia. Previous ministerial task force reports had argued that the fundamental problem with Nova Scotia's health care system was excessive centralization. The 1989 Gallant report had asserted that "[t]he current centralized administration of the health care system inhibits meaningful local and regional participation of citizens and health care providers in the planning and management of health care resources" (Nova Scotia, 1989, 12), and suggested that "[a] decentralized and rationalized process of decision-making should result in effective and efficient use of existing capital" (15). The 1994 report had reinforced this position, arguing that provincial control over the four regional health boards was too stringent, and would lead to a "rigid, inflexible, and unresponsive" form of centralized control (Nova Scotia, 1994, 6). Based on these analyses, Nova Scotia's health system was reorganized to accommodate a more dispersed regional framework; and in 2001 nine discrete district health authorities were established in place of the four regional health authorities (Figure 7.1). Informed by the school of New Public Management, this approach was premised on the principle that managerial units more closely situated in the community were better able to utilize available resources in a way that was more responsive to the needs of the local population.

Formally, these regional units were responsible for the delivery of services, while the provincial Department of Health focused on the strategic direction of health planning, as well as the allocation of budgets for each of the regional units. The minister of health retained responsibility for the "development, implementation, and evaluation" of health policy; the development of standards for health care delivery; monitoring, measuring, and evaluating the quality, accessibility, and comprehensiveness of health services; financial and human resources planning; and establishing the requirements for information systems. The minister could

Figure 7.1 Map of district health authorities in Nova Scotia, 2001–15

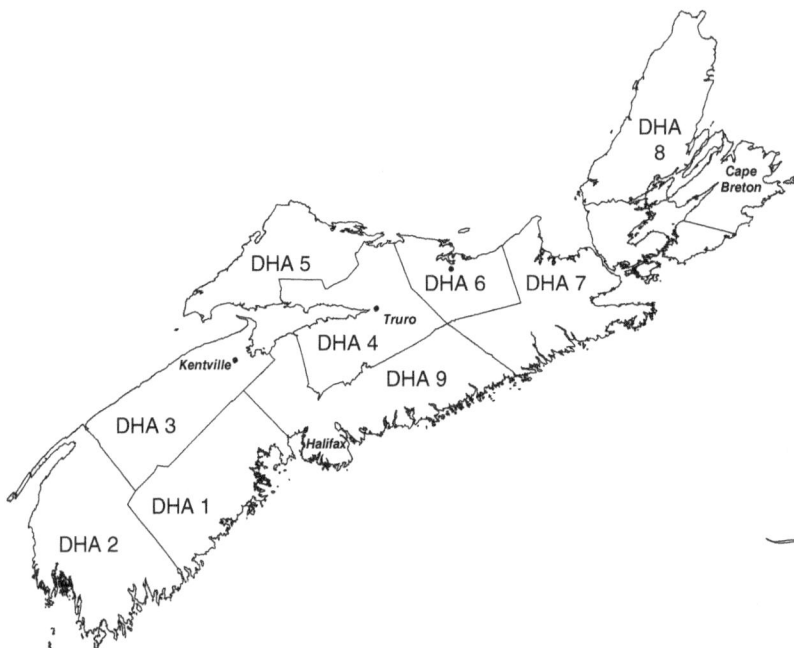

also place "binding directions" on the DHAs on any matter the minister considered relevant. The province retained oversight of nine independent programs focusing on cancer care, diabetes, cardiovascular health, organ donation, kidney disease, breast cancer screening, blood collection, reproductive care, and hearing and speech. These programs set standards and monitored coordination in each of their respective areas; some, though not all, provided services directly. As the DHAs provided most of the delivery of services that addressed these conditions (cancer care, diabetes care, mental health care, etc.), these programs worked informally with the DHAs (including funding discrete projects under the programs' purview) respecting the objectives specified by their mandates. However, there were no formal direct relationships between the nine provincial programs and the DHAs (Figure 7.2).

The narrative of health care reorganization in Nova Scotia under the 2013 Liberal administration is interwoven tightly with provincial labour relations, and it is worth focusing on this in some detail. The "policy window" for health care reform in 2013 was situated in a sense of urgency

Figure 7.2 Organizational chart of the Nova Scotia health system prior to 2015 reform

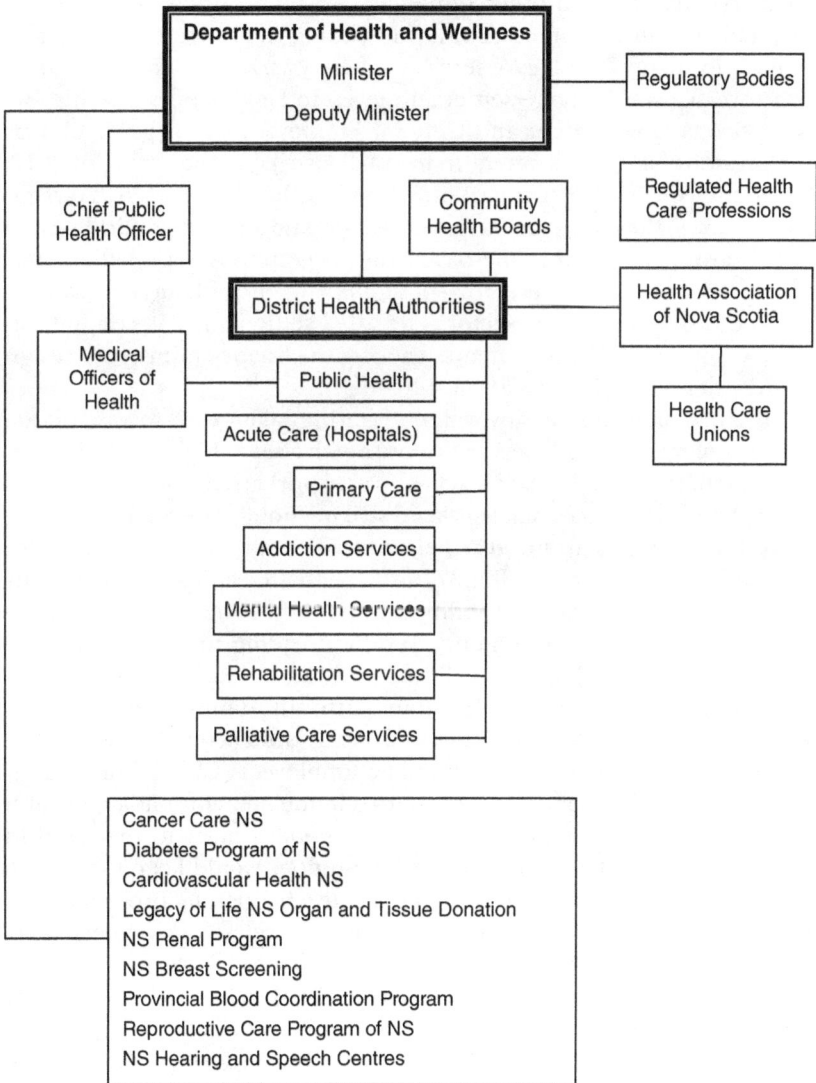

Department of Health and Wellness
Minister
Deputy Minister

Regulatory Bodies

Regulated Health Care Professions

Chief Public Health Officer

Community Health Boards

District Health Authorities

Health Association of Nova Scotia

Medical Officers of Health

Public Health

Health Care Unions

Acute Care (Hospitals)

Primary Care

Addiction Services

Mental Health Services

Rehabilitation Services

Palliative Care Services

Cancer Care NS
Diabetes Program of NS
Cardiovascular Health NS
Legacy of Life NS Organ and Tissue Donation
NS Renal Program
NS Breast Screening
Provincial Blood Coordination Program
Reproductive Care Program of NS
NS Hearing and Speech Centres

that arose from the recognition that Nova Scotia was spending the high-est proportion of the provincial budget on health care (47 per cent in 2013) compared to all other Canadian provinces. It was compounded by public dissatisfaction at also having among the longest wait times in Canada for many health care services. There was, at the same time, some controversy over the large settlement given to Halifax nurses within the Nova Scotia Government and General Employees Union (NSGEU) by the previous NDP government to forestall a strike in the spring of 2012. While the NSGEU represented only 2,547 of the province's 6,726 regis-tered nurses, they were an extremely well-organized and politically com-mitted group, and had in the past achieved generous wage settlements, which then set the pattern for subsequent wage settlements through-out the province's public sector. The 2012 settlement was contentious even within the NDP government, causing the finance minister to resign shortly thereafter (Steele, 2014a, 146–9).

The incoming Liberal government, having taken care to win a large majority of seats in 2013, began its tenure with a set of high-profile labour-relations bills directed squarely at health care workers. Bill 30, the Essential Home Support Services Act, legislated striking home care workers back to work. The bill was introduced 28 February 2014 and was given royal assent one day later, on March 1. Bill 37, the Essential Health and Community Services Act, constrained the ability of nurses and other health care work-ers to strike. This bill, too, went from first reading to royal assent in 2 days. The premier's popularity did not fall but rather increased notably over this period (Angus Reid Institute, 2016). In August 2014 the largest health care union, the NSGEU, as well as the Nova Scotia Nurses' Union (NSNU), the Canadian Union of Public Employees (CUPE), and Unifor requested that the unions be represented in the new consolidated health authority within a bargaining-association model similar to that used in British Columbia. Under this model, the unions would keep their exist-ing members and, at the start of any collective bargaining process, would form a bargaining association comprising the relevant members (e.g., nurses) from any of the existing unions. This model was, in principle, the structure that was ultimately established in March 2015. However, the government strenuously resisted this option throughout the 6 months of negotiation over the consolidation of the health authorities; and a discus-sion of the nature of these negotiations illustrates the close association between health care reorganization and labour relations in Nova Scotia.

In September 2014, Minister of Health and Wellness Leo Glavine rejected the unions' request for a bargaining-association model, stating that "it has not adequately addressed valid and significant concerns articulated by the employer representatives, nor has it resolved all of the issues of interest for this government" (CBC, 2014b). Bill One, the Health Authorities Act 2014, was introduced by the government on 29 September 2014. By October 3, it had gone through first reading, second reading, the law amendments committee, third reading, and royal assent. What was notable in the legislation was the process governing the restructuring of bargaining units. Citing the difficulty of bargaining on an ongoing basis with more than 50 different units, the province introduced a provision in Bill One that would categorize all health care workers into four discrete groups: nursing, clerical, health care, and support workers. In the past, when functional units were merged due to administrative reorganization in Nova Scotia, the practice had normally been to hold runoff votes within each bargaining unit to determine which unit would represent workers in the collective bargaining process. While this usual procedure could have achieved the government's stated objective of rationalizing the bargaining process, the province insisted that it had the authority arbitrarily to assign all health care workers to the union of its own choosing. Many commentators saw this as an attempt by the government to "kneecap" the influential NSGEU to prevent it from establishing generous settlements across the public sector (Steele, 2015).

Under the terms of the new Health Authorities Act 2014, a mediator-arbitrator (James Dorsey) was selected in October 2014 to work out the details regarding which workers would be classified into which category, and which union would then represent each of the four new groups. In the mediation phase of this process, it became clear that the positions of the government and the unions were quite far apart in process as well as in substance. The government's representative in the negotiations, the Health Association of Nova Scotia (HANS), maintained that the role of the mediator-arbitrator was simply to interpret and apply the new statute, while the unions argued that the law contravened the right to freedom of association protected by the Charter of Rights and Freedoms. On 18 November, it became clear that the mediation phase had failed, and the negotiations went into the arbitration phase on 9 December 2014.

Dorsey presented his arbitration report on 17 January 2015. It was generally expected that the report would constitute an end to the process, but the report was remarkably open-ended in its assessment. The report achieved a key technical objective in classifying all of the province's health care workers into the four categories specified by the Health Authorities Act. It also declared that the legislation did not violate the

Charter provision for freedom of association in requiring health care workers to belong to a bargaining unit based on their job classification *as long as* the government did not arbitrarily determine the representation of each of these groups. Dorsey's report stressed the critical importance of the principle of majoritarianism, and it queried how a collective agreement could be considered valid and enforceable if the union chosen did not represent a majority of the employees (Dorsey, 2015). In this way the government was informed that it did not have the authority to impose a bargaining agent on a group of employees represented by a different union. This point was reinforced by two decisions released by the Supreme Court of Canada in January 2015 supporting unions' freedom of association (*Mounted Police Association of Ontario v. Canada [Attorney General]*, 2015 SCC 1 and *Saskatchewan Federation of Labour v. Saskatchewan*, 2015 SCC 4). Rather than imposing a final settlement in his January report, Dorsey encouraged the parties to come to more "creative solutions" to break the impasse and rejected the government's call that his role was simply to interpret and apply the statute:

> The Mediator-Arbitrator is not simply an usher showing everyone pre-assigned seating. The Mediator-Arbitrator is not simply a facilitator clearing the field and setting up for a new game that has a new player in the mix with old players assigned new positions. The Mediator-Arbitrator's role is not simply to ensure the employers or the government gets a desired outcome, no matter how much it might be preordained. (ibid.)

Another blow to the government was Dorsey's ruling that all categories of workers, to be legitimate, had to comprise a majority in *each* of the two health authorities (NSHA and IWK). Only one union – the NSGEU – had a double majority in any of the four areas; and thus Dorsey awarded representation of health care workers to the NSGEU. Under this principle, the NSNU, which was expected to represent all nurses, fell short of a double majority. The arbitrator had declared that licensed practical nurses were to be represented in the same unit as registered nurses and, when they were added to the calculation, the NSNU's double majority no longer existed. The government retorted that it would use the regulations set out in the new Health Authorities Act to redefine, through orders in council, how licensed practical nurses would be classified, thereby ensuring that the NSNU would be granted representation of the nurses. In a second ruling, on 19 February 2015, Dorsey pointed out that the government's authority to impose regulations under the act did not actually come into effect until 1 April 2015, when the act itself took effect; and that such an attempt arbitrarily to define one of the classifications through regulations imposed through orders in council would thus be inconsistent with the law. The 19 February report also noted that were two NSGEU locals to merge, the NSGEU would then have a double majority respecting another category: clerical workers. If the merger were to be completed before a stipulated date, said Dorsey, the NSGEU would thus be able to represent a second category of workers.

The Nova Scotia government immediately issued a press release in which the health minister stated that "Mr. Dorsey was given a clear mandate: to create a labour landscape that would allow the changes Nova Scotians know are needed. He has failed to fulfill his mandate" (Nova Scotia Department of Health and Wellness, 2015c). The minister rejected the February ruling and declared that the province would introduce legislation to determine which union would represent the three remaining bargaining units. When the NSGEU merger of clerical workers' unions was completed on 25 February 2015, Dorsey formally recognized the NSGEU as the new bargaining agent for the clerical workers, despite claims by the government that he had already been fired. The CBC, which had been keeping track of the correspondence from the government to Dorsey, noted that the mediator-arbitrator had been fired three times in 2 days (four times, if a phone call were added to written dismissals) (CBC, 2015). There was considerable discussion as to whether the government was legally able to "fire" Dorsey at all given the terms of his contract. Regardless of this debate, the NSGEU immediately registered Dorsey's 25 February decision as an order of the court, thereby ensuring that it had a binding effect in law. For the government to rescind the order, it would have to do so through a legislative act in a full sitting of the Legislative Assembly.

On 3 March 2015, the premier took over the file from the health minister and, in the spirit of Dorsey's suggestion to engage in "creative solutions," invited all four unions to a process of confidential negotiation. The premier announced on 13 March that a deal had been reached. Under the terms of this agreement, each union retained its original membership. For purposes of negotiation and for the administration of the collective agreements, new bodies ("Councils") comprised the relevant members of each existing union (Figure 7.3). The NSNU would lead negotiations for the nurses across both health authorities (in the Nova Scotia Council of Nursing Unions); the NSGEU would lead for the health-care workers (in the Nova Scotia Council of Health Care Unions);

Figure 7.3 Composition of the new health authority bargaining units (nurses)

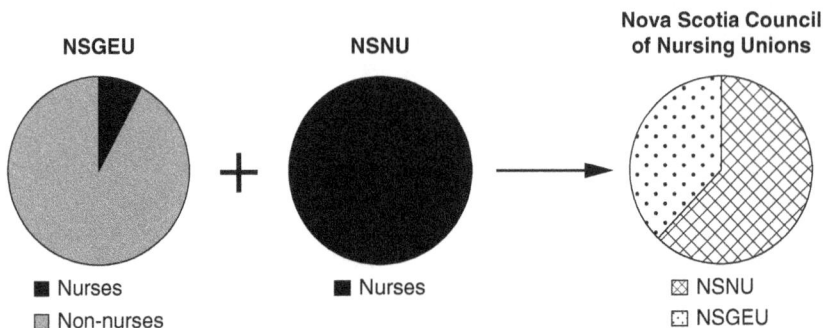

CUPE would lead for the clerical workers (in the Nova Scotia Council of Health Administrative Professional Unions); and Unifor would lead for support workers (in the Nova Scotia Council of Health Support Unions). These new associations were recognized in the Health Authorities Act through an amendment (Bill 69), and they were formally certified as bargaining agents by the Nova Scotia Labour Board on 8 April 2015.

The narrative of events surrounding the reclassification and representation of health care workers within the new system of health governance does not imply that reorganization was undertaken solely to undermine the influence of strong unions. But given that the consolidation of unions *could* have been accomplished in a more neutral and disengaged manner, it does suggest that the reorganization was nonetheless seen as an opportunity to diminish the influence of key unions. The government's health reform strategy has consistently been interconnected with its labour relations strategy, although it is unclear how closely one is dependent on the other. To the extent that the wages and salaries of health care workers are a large component of health care costs, and given that the new NSHA is committed to achieving a balanced budget (Nova Scotia Health Authority, 2015a), the focus on wage settlements for health care workers is perhaps unsurprising.

The Nova Scotia Health Authority came into being on 1 April 2015. But the government was not finished with its labour legislation. In December 2015 the government introduced Bill 148, the Public Services Sustainability Act. This bill legislated a wage pattern for public sector workers of 0, 0, 1, 1.5, and 0.5 per cent over several years. Arbitrators involved in collective bargaining negotiations would under the legislation be limited in the amounts that they would be able to award. However, the bill remained "contingent on proclamation," which meant that the government passed it while the legislature was sitting but would bring it into force only if negotiations with public sector unions broke down and put the government's fiscal objectives at risk.

It is worth reiterating here, following the analysis of Lazar et al. (2013), that the substantial reforms being made by the Nova Scotia government during this period were administrative rather than programmatic. They did not incorporate changes that affected health care users directly. Demand-based health care reform (getting patients to use fewer or less expensive goods or services) was a cost-reduction strategy that the government did not pursue. This was likely a calculated political choice. As a former Nova Scotia MLA remarked, "[m]essing up health issues may well lose a government voter support (and this is always a risk for a government and not so much for an opposition). But competent delivery of the services does not usually attract votes. Competent delivery is what voters expect as a given" (Epstein, 2015, 100).

7.2 The reorganization of the Department of Health and Wellness

Before consolidating its health authorities, the province of Nova Scotia consulted at length with other provinces that had attempted similar initiatives (especially Alberta). A key lesson that Nova Scotia distilled from these experiences, and from previous attempts at regionalization, was that any undertaking to change the configuration of district health authorities would be undermined by an ossified departmental structure that had evolved to support the previous governance system. Provinces that had undertaken systematic changes to their system of regionalization had never restructured their departments of health to support the new configuration: Nova Scotia, in contrast, would reorganize its health department to facilitate the administrative redesign of its health authority structure.

Prior to the 2015 consolidation of nine DHAs to one, key functions of the DHW included coordinating activity across the DHAs and providing a general direction to (and oversight of) programs and services offered at the DHA level. The principle underlying regionalization was that each DHA was responsible for the delivery of health care services at the regional level. When regionalization was introduced in the mid-1990s, hospital-based services and programs were amalgamated within regional health authorities, but the decision-making process was still understood to be responsive to local needs and concerns because of the regional administrative structure. This meant a bifurcated focus on many major programs at both the regional and provincial level. These included mental health, children's services, addiction services, cancer care, and continuing care, which required province-wide standards and processes. These services were provided and funded at the regional level, but the DHW monitored and evaluated these programs on an ongoing basis. It attempted to ensure that accessibility remained reasonably uniform between regions and demographic groups. The province also set the priorities that DHAs were expected to recognize and determined the allocation of funding for these programs.

The DHW also addressed several functions that were more specific to centralized administrative control. It performed a complex coordination function, harmonizing the activity between government departments (including Community Services, Justice, and Education); between provincial departments and DHAs; between other community agencies and NGOs; and (especially in the areas of long-term care and home case) with private providers. The DHW also focused on broader issues such as workforce planning (including recruitment and retention, education and training, and compensation); pharmaceutical services (generally for seniors and lower-income individuals); and financial planning (including funding models for provider organizations, investment in capital infrastructure; forecasting, procurement, and internal audits). As information systems became an ever more integral aspect of health care services, the province also established the province-wide requirements for IT systems, not only for electronic health records, but also for the collection of data and the use of this data in addressing issues such as patient safety and wait times. Another major function of the DHW was public health. This not only focused on communicable disease prevention, but also on complex nonmedical determinants of health, disease surveillance, and emergency preparedness and response (see Figure 7.4).

The consolidation of nine DHAs into the NSHA meant that the coordinating function of the DHW became largely irrelevant. The restructuring of the DHA system thus required the DHW's internal organization to be reconfigured to reflect the new provincial structure. In January 2016, the provincial government announced its changes to the DHW. These came into effect in April 2016. The most apparent change was that the duplication of services at the regional and provincial levels was eliminated. All responsibility for acute and tertiary care, mental health and addictions, primary health care, health system quality, and some physician services now resides directly with the NSHA. Public health is now under the aegis of the NSHA, although the chief medical officer of health still reports directly to the deputy minister. Two portfolios remain with the province. The first is clinical IT applications, which primarily focuses

Figure 7.4 Internal organization chart of the Department of Health and Wellness prior to 2016

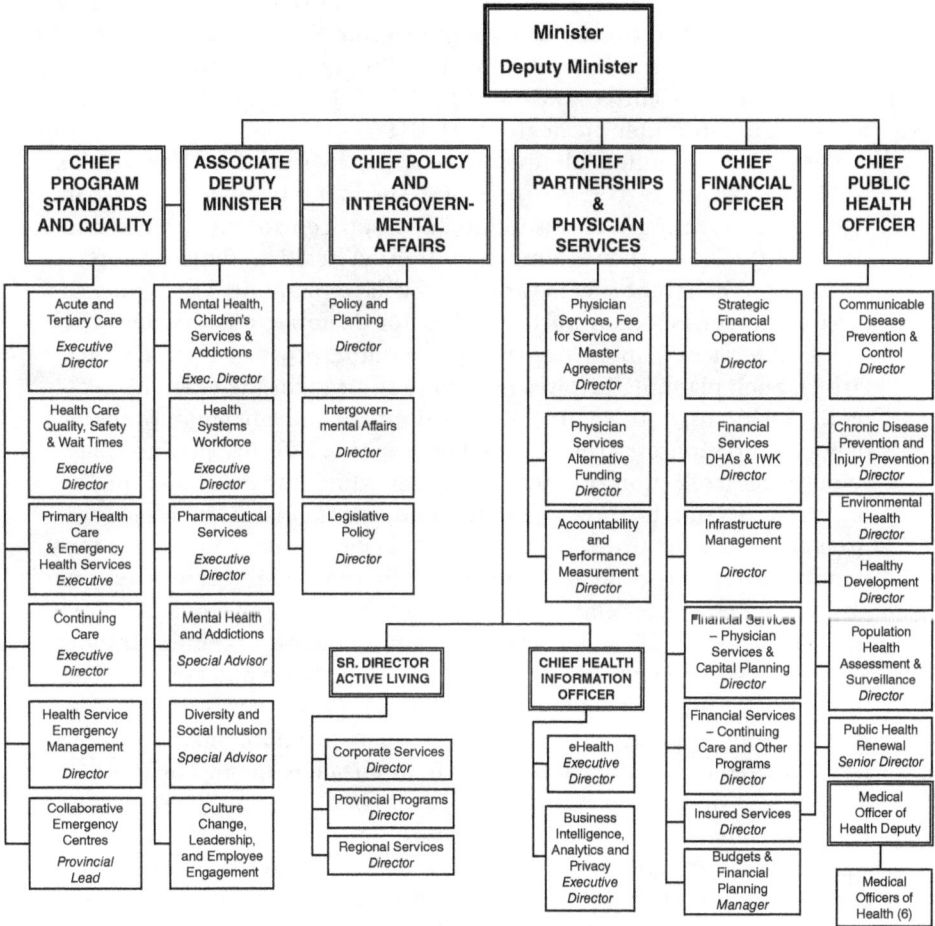

Source: Government of Nova Scotia, Management Guide (http://www.novascotia.ca/treasuryboard /manuals/PDF/100/H&W.pdf).

on the development of the "One Person, One Record" electronic health system. The second is continuing care. A related change was the transfer of six of the nine discrete programs from provincial authority to the NSHA. These programs are relatively self-governing and generally have governance structures involving boards of directors or advisory councils.

The six programs transferred to the NSHA are Cancer Care NS, Diabetes Care NS, Cardiovascular Health NS, the NS Organ and Tissue Donation Program (Legacy of Life); NS Provincial Blood Coordinating Program, and the NS Renal Program. Two programs (the Reproductive Care Program of NS and the NS Breast Screening Program) were transferred to the IWK Health Centre; and one (the Hearing and Speech Program) remains directly under the aegis of the DHW.

The transfer of much administrative authority from the DHW to the NSHA has created two types of tensions. The first is the tension between regional and central administration (i.e., between the new zones and the NSHA). On one hand, a more centralized health authority can provide a more coherent system-wide approach to planning. One concern driving the consolidation of the DHAs, for example, was the need for a clinical-services plan encompassing the entire province (Nova Scotia, 2014f). Such planning involves not only a strategy for the efficient treatment of patients, but also the bulk procurement and efficient movement of goods and services across regional boundaries. Effective planning also requires the collection of information regarding outcomes and quality of care across the regions: and, to this end, the standardization of measurement across the province more easily facilitates the data required to establish any strategic plan. A more centralized administrative system also facilitates greater standardization in programs and services across the province. On the other hand, the consolidation of administration also raises issues about the loss of local representation and control. The imposition of uniform benchmarks by its very nature may be disadvantageous to some regions, either by showing them in a poor light, or simply by failing to measure or facilitate what is important to them. The move to standardization also meant that some areas could lose specific programs that were *superior* to those offered across the province. The zonal model was obviously an attempt to establish a midway representational structure that would enable the NSHA to recognize and understand "what is needed at a local level" (ibid., 8). However, *hearing* local voices is not necessarily the same as *responding* to them. In terms of local representation, a great deal will depend on how much decision-making authority the new zones have. A regional hospital that has to go farther up the decision-making ladder than before to effect desired changes will not be convinced that a centralized governance structure is more "efficient."

A second tension in the new organizational scheme is the issue of relative autonomy between the NSHA and the DHW. The stated advantage of having a comprehensive managerial unit separate from the DHW is that the health authority can attend to the daily operational issues at a systemic level, while the health department can focus more fully on setting strategic policy directions. In practice, however, this distinction is considerably more blurred. The NSHA, for example, has been directed not only to follow through on strategic planning as articulated by the DHW, but also to develop "important initiatives" with "a commitment to innovation" (Nova Scotia Health Authority, 2015a). What is not clear is how effectively it will be able to do so at one remove from the legislative and policy tools available to the DHW (which can, for example, mandate through legislation that particular actions are executed, or coordinate activity between departments, or represent the province in intergovernmental fora).

A related governance issue is the monitoring and evaluation of quality and performance. Prior to the 2016 reforms, the Quality and Patient Safety branch within the DHW was responsible for quality standards and safety improvement. In 2016 this function was transferred to the NSHA. This move facilitated the standardization of data collection essential to measuring and evaluating performance across a system (e.g., in the reporting of outcomes). Yet it also permits the NSHA to police itself in the identification, reporting, and correction of safety and quality problems. One question that arises here is whether self-monitoring is the most conducive means of assuring transparency and accountability in the system, or whether independent oversight is more effective. Another question is how the evaluation and monitoring of services *outside* of the NSHA (e.g., in continuing-care facilities) will be assured. The minister has stated that "it will be the department that will have final oversight" (Gorman, 2016b), but it is unclear precisely how this oversight will manifest itself (e.g., whether any accountability issues that arise in services outside the NSHA and addressed directly by the province will be made available for public scrutiny). Similarly, if the DHW chooses to micromanage small but politically intense situations that arise in the NSHA, then the very point of having an independent health authority is rather undermined.

7.3 Summary

The organizational reforms executed in 2015 and 2016 amount to a considerable change in the way health care is administered in Nova Scotia. The consolidation of nine health authorities into a single entity and the transfer of competencies from the DHW to the new NSHA potentially gives the new health authority significant scope to effect further reforms and refinements. A key component of this new focus will be capacity building. Nova Scotia has some difficulty in accessing its data efficiently enough to be able to develop well-considered evidence-based strategic planning. A more integrated and system-wide approach to data collection and access is a useful starting point. In February 2016, the minister noted that the DHW was working to create a quality health council (Gorman, 2016b), although no specifics were given.

The reforms may facilitate the development of health-related IT systems across the province (such as One Person, One Record). A more central focus can also clarify issues of access and service eligibility between regions, and it can permit the utilization of health care resources across boundaries in a more efficient manner. At the same time, however, the new administrative structure confronts a largely rural (and increasingly depopulated) constituency that expects a voice in resource allocation and program development even as scale economies in the provision of care in these areas become more difficult to achieve. Likewise, establishing a new administrative entity with greater authority will remove many obstacles to the development and implementation of policy solutions for specific problems. But the lack of clear oversight mechanisms raises the question of how accountability will be allocated if and when problems arise. Moreover, the hard line taken by the province against health care workers has led to an atmosphere that is not particularly conducive to negotiating innovative new delivery systems. The reforms enacted in 2015 and 2016 have a great deal of potential but, as with any new policy direction, they will have to navigate around pitfalls both predictable and unanticipated.

Chapter Eight

Assessment of the Health System

The assessment of any health care system depends a great deal on our understanding of what we expect it to do. Across Canada, as elsewhere, the goal is to improve the experience of care, advance the health of populations, and reduce per capita costs of health care (Berwick, Nolan, & Whittington, 2008). A high-performing health care system should be able to provide safe and effective health services and should do so in a manner that is "patient-centred" (Stewart, 2001). This means, among other things, that patients are treated respectfully; that they are given a sense of agency in choosing treatment options; that these treatments reflect the values and priorities held by patients; and that, at a system level, all the different services patients may require are well-coordinated and easily navigated. A high-performing health care system should also provide comprehensive services: this not only means that appropriate services exist, but also that they can be accessed without undue barriers, such as cost or waiting time. Barriers to access can also be influenced by age, gender, race, language, sexual orientation, disability, or geography (e.g., Bowen, 2001; Mathieson, Bailey, & Gurevich, 2002; Hajizadeh, 2017). This is particularly important in a country such as Canada, where equity in health care provision is widely supported (Galloway, 2016). Another important, though more complicated, measure of assessment is the extent to which potential health conditions are prevented from developing in the first place. "Upstream" factors such as education, nutrition, physical fitness, income, housing, and freedom from undue mental or physical adversity can all play a role in keeping populations healthy (Williams, Costa, Odunlami, & Mohammed, 2008); but because distinct and measureable causal relationships are difficult to ascertain conclusively, the link between these nonmedical determinants of health and the overall health of a society can be difficult to evaluate (Braveman, Egerter, Woolf, & Marks, 2011).

Nova Scotia's formal health care goals are articulated in the Department of Health and Wellness's annual statements of mandate and focus on economic stewardship, the health of the population, experience of care, and health workforce. These categories are discussed in more detail below. There are two particular difficulties in assessing the Nova Scotia health care system. The first is the lack of a robust set of key public performance indicators and longitudinal data to assess the extent of progress across the health care sector over time. In 2016, the Department of Health and Wellness (DHW) introduced an accountability framework that could allow such assessments to take place in the future; at present, this data is still limited and uneven. The second problem is in assessing the reforms themselves. The aim of the reforms executed in 2015 and 2016 was to distinguish clearly between policy development and evaluation (performed by the DHW) and health services delivery (under the purview of the Nova Scotia Health Authority [NSHA]). Governance structures were redesigned to permit a "more streamlined, cost-effective system" to stimulate innovation, facilitate access to care, and improve health outcomes (Nova Scotia Health Authority, 2015a).

Yet, as Savoie (2015) cautions, the articulation of new policy design is easy enough; the real test is whether or not a government is able effectively to implement it. It is difficult to evaluate major reforms while the dust is still settling. Nonetheless, it is useful to parse in more detail the advantages identified by the architects of the new reforms: it is noteworthy, for example, that a more consolidated governance system is being propounded for its capacity for greater innovation (Nova Scotia Health Authority, 2015a, 2), given the essential insight of New Public Management that centralization was generally responsible for *stifling* innovation. This is especially important when political agents implement structural reforms that are founded on a very limited evidence base (Marchildon, 2015, 2016). It is therefore useful, as Hassenteufel et al. (2010) and Marmor and Wendt (2012) argue, to employ an actor-centred approach to health policy change, and to identify *who* promotes any particular policy direction, *how* they intend to execute it, and *why* they chose to do so. The political explanations for reforms, they note, are often as significant as the stated policy objectives themselves.

The development of organizational frameworks for the administration of health are as much about shifting the relationships of power and influence as they are about program delivery and cost-effectiveness (Fierlbeck,

2016). And from this perspective, the trend towards the amalgamation of health regions can be seen as a logical extension of the previous wave of health care regionalization. One of the initial objectives of regionalization was to diminish the opportunity for capture by provider interests at a local (hospital board) level. In the same way, small health regions "with fewer resources and with boards whose members are more personally connected to their community" have been less resistant to clientelism (Lomas, 2003, 356); and amalgamation into larger administrative units was seen as a means of curtailing local provider capture. Duckett, for example, documents how regionalized health care in Alberta was "often seen as part of local wealth creation, with local employment prioritized over system efficiency and more contemporary service delivery modes and local procurement used to support local providers" (2015, 321). Rather than representing an about-face in policy direction, then, the amalgamation of health regions into a single authority is merely the extension of what has been a steady process of disengaging local interests from capturing service provision. Yet such a strategy is not without its own risks. As Duckett argues, a single health authority faces its own challenges, including a different kind of diseconomies of scale (such as multiple layers of reporting); the removal of top decision makers from local communities, leading to diminished local responsiveness; the disruption of local coordination; and the potential that a single authority can lose its independence to a "micro-managing minister" (2016, 56). When the dust settles on Nova Scotia's administrative reforms, then, any evaluation of the effectiveness of these reforms will have address not only traditional health and health system indicators, but also whether the structural changes have been able to avoid these potential political pitfalls.

8.1 The province's strategic goals

8.1.1 Resource stewardship

A key objective of the new system is the attainment of a "sustainable" and "fiscally responsible" health care system (Nova Scotia Department of Health and Wellness, 2015d). Reflecting this priority, the new NSHA in its first business plan committed itself to achieving a balanced budget (Nova Scotia Health Authority, 2015a). This was, to a large extent, to be accomplished through the "leaning of administrative roles" in the health care system (ibid., 7). It is difficult, without a financial audit, to determine whether, or to what extent, "administrative efficiency" has been achieved through the consolidation of district health authorities (DHAs). The NSHA projected savings of $41,584,039 in 2015–16; $6,210,000 of this was to be from "salary and compensation savings related to DHA executive restructuring" (ibid., appendix B). However, the document did not provide a detailed breakdown of how and where these cost savings would arise. Nor did it include the severance payments to administrators who were laid off, which were estimated to be $4.8 million. A FOI request reported in the Halifax *Chronicle Herald* also showed that the province incurred an additional $3.7 million for merging computerized financial systems across the former DHAs. The total merger cost was estimated in 2015 to be nine million dollars (Gorman, 2015).

There is little hard evidence that administrative rationalization has resulted in cost savings in the short term. The difficulty with much health reform is that it is often necessary to spend money in the short run to save money in the long term. It is certainly arguable that a consolidated administrative structure can facilitate a more efficient operating system, as it permits easier transfer of goods and services across regional boundaries and supports the development of information systems needed to evaluate system-wide performance. But these are largely long-term savings; and the longer the time frame, the more difficult it is precisely to identify and compare the hypothetical costs that *would* have been incurred in the path *not* taken. Even before the amalgamation took effect, the individual tasked with supervising the merger acknowledged that "there would likely be no savings in the initial years of the merger but rather later into the process" (Gorman, 2014). The minister of health and wellness admitted that the electoral campaign claim stating that the reorganization would lead to savings of $13 million per year was perhaps "oversimplified," and that it wasn't clear to him before arriving at the DHW that the election promise "probably wasn't doable": "That will be there, but it's just going to take a longer path to get there. That's what I realize as health minister now" (ibid.).

The advantages of running a balanced health care budget are fairly straightforward; the sustainability of a health care system over the long term does in the end depend on having the resources to fund it. Yet committing politically to a balanced budget in health care can present serious problems as well. The physical infrastructure supporting Nova Scotia's health care system, as the auditor general noted on more than one occasion, is in perilous disrepair. The DHW has known of the state of decline for some time. The Victoria General Hospital in Halifax, in particular, came under a great deal of public scrutiny in 2015, when water pipes burst, flooding several floors of the hospital, and again in 2016, when photos of dilapidated rooms were widely posted on social media. Yet successive governments were unwilling directly to address the issue of replacing this facility, given the estimated $1.3 billion replacement cost. No governments in recent decades in Nova Scotia have been willing to sanction deficit financing over several election cycles, and major capital projects threatening the balanced-budget position of any governing administration have simply been pushed to the side. The commitment to avoid deficits can provide the impetus to operational efficiency in the short term, but it can also seriously undermine system integrity over the long run. For example, a balanced health care budget was achieved in the 2015–16 fiscal year, but only because of delays in capital construction, delays in IT projects, program delays, decreased utilization of vaccine programs, and decreased spending in Primary Health Renewal and physician services despite a serious shortage of doctors in the province (Nova Scotia 2016b, 56).

8.1.2 Health of the population

With a higher proportion of older adults and higher rates of chronic disease compared to most other Canadian provinces, Nova Scotia must focus steadily on care for the elderly, primary health care, and health promotion. As in other jurisdictions, progress in these policy areas is slow and often intractable. The province has been able to make a slight reduction in waitlists for long-term care but, as chapter 4 notes, this was largely through revising the way in which waitlists were determined. One option for the province to provide home care and long-term care more inexpensively would be through a process of tendering. This strategy, however, has been firmly rebuffed by care recipients, who argue that it would be detrimental to the quality of care received, and by care providers, who believe that it would mean lower wages for them. Tendering systems have also not provided simple solutions for problems faced by home care programs in other jurisdictions. The dementia strategy and palliative care strategy introduced by the province may have some effect on addressing care for the elderly, but both are in early stages of development.

Chronic disease is another source of major health expenditure for the province. The top 1 per cent of health care users in Nova Scotia between 2010 and 2012 accounted for 33.4 per cent of total physician and inpatient hospital costs, while 5 per cent accounted for 63.8 per cent (mainly in the form of inpatient hospitalization). Health expenditure is to a large extent directed to a very small number of individuals, but these individuals often present multiple and complex chronic conditions, such as heart and respiratory disease, diabetes, and mental illness. In Nova Scotia, more than three-quarters of high-resource users have two or more of these conditions, while a quarter have four or more. For high users, diabetes is the disease with the highest prevalence, followed by respiratory disease (predominantly COPD), and then heart disease. It is interesting to note that while both diabetes and cardiovascular health have discrete programs dedicated to addressing these diseases, there is no similar program for respiratory disease (all data Kephart et al., 2016). The high rate of chronic disease also requires a systematic attempt to prevent chronic illnesses before they arise. The province's main health promotion program, "Thrive!," attempts to provide lifestyle advice, planning, and opportunities for children and families, although there has been little evaluation of the effectiveness of this program (Nova Scotia, 2014e).

8.1.3 Appropriate, good-quality care

The province's strategy to provide cost-effective, good-quality health care services has two components. The first is the move towards collaborative primary care. There has been clear progress on some aspects of this strategy. There has been a substantial increase in the number of primary health care interdisciplinary teams in the province in the past decade. The development of collaborative emergency centres, in particular, in a number of locations across the province has established a template for the way in which health care providers can work in a way that best utilizes the competencies of each profession in rural areas. From a regulatory perspective, the Regulated Health Professions Network Act provides a flexible regulatory structure for collaborative engagement by all regulated health care professionals.

At the same time, however, it has been difficult to move many GP practices to a broader, more collaborative model that provides weekend and after-hours services to patients. Here, the major reforms in health care restructuring in Nova Scotia have not been particularly helpful. In the first place, physicians' accountability to the NSHA remains unclear. What is it, specifically, that the health authority is purchasing from them? Nova Scotia has been more successful in moving away from a fee-for-service system; almost half the province's physicians are remunerated on alternative payment plans (CIHI, 2015b, 10). But these payments are often based on a confusing mix of services rendered (inputs) and outcomes (outputs) and are not particularly well monitored or evaluated (Nova Scotia Office of the Auditor General, 2014b). More troubling from an organizational perspective is that under the new provincial reforms, the responsibility for the management of physicians is very unclear. As chapter 2 outlines, the new NSHA (specifically, the VP medicine and

integrated health services) is responsible for physician services (physician performance evaluation, credentialing, resources planning, and
remuneration). Nonetheless, the province itself is directly responsible for
negotiating the Master Agreement with physicians. The problem is that
substantial changes to the primary health system (such as the development
of more collaborative, interdisciplinary health care teams) will depend on
implementing effective team-based funding models, which can be negotiated only through the physicians' Master Agreement. It is thus difficult to
see how the NSHA can move ahead with more effective primary health
care reforms without the direct involvement of the DHW (and vice versa).

Another aspect of the strategy to achieve "appropriate, good quality
care" is an "increased emphasis upon evidence and data to inform planning and system learning to improve safety and service delivery" (Nova
Scotia Department of Health and Wellness, 2015d, 8). What this statement leaves unsaid is the lack of effective information systems on which
to base planning and system learning. To an extent, this was precisely
one of the objectives of consolidating the DHAs. But it will be a gradual process. There are some specialized information systems currently
in place: wait times are monitored and posted by the Patient Access
Registry; patient safety incidents are tracked and reported through the
Safety Improvement and Management System; and surgical services are
evaluated through the Provincial Perioperative Advisory Committee. But
much of the analytical information needed to provide "evidence-based"
services by assessing how well programs work is still lacking. The new
Health Authorities Act requires the development of a health services
plan to establish "what services should be offered in the health system,
where those services should be provided, and by who[m]" (ibid.). This
plan will be complemented by the implementation of the National Surgical Quality Improvement Program in both the NSHA and the IWK.

8.1.4 Health system workforce

The fourth key objective in the province's health care strategy is the
development of a finely calibrated workforce. This requires a close monitoring of the supply of, and demand for, all health care professionals.
The province must be able to discern how many individuals in each profession are licensed and active in the province, how many are scheduled
to retire, where are they practising, and how their skills are being used.
The goal is to identify "the right number, mix, and distribution" of
health care providers throughout the province. This policy objective also

requires a focus on the recruitment and retention of health care professionals. To this end, Nova Scotia has developed and refined a needs-
based nursing strategy and a physician resources planning document to
assist in the provision of the requisite health workers across the province. Yet the DHW does not systematically evaluate how service providers
are performing in areas such as nursing homes (Nova Scotia Office of
the Auditor General, 2016a, 15). In some cases, the contracts for services providers themselves do not specify performance evaluations and
reporting provisions; in other cases, where these are specified, there is
little follow-up to determine whether expectations were met.

At the same time, the province's relationship with both public- and private-sector workers has been severely strained by acrimonious negotiation
and divisive labour relations legislation enacted between 2014 and 2016.
The physicians' Master Agreement, for example, which expired in March
2015, failed to be renegotiated for over a year; many physicians were being
reimbursed through alternative funding plans that had expired several
years previously. A Master Agreement is normally a complex document
to negotiate, but the process was made considerably more difficult by the
passage of Nova Scotia's wage restraint legislation, which barred physicians access to arbitration over pay disputes. A new Master Agreement was
finally ratified in June 2016, though physicians remain dissatisfied at the
lack of input they have in health policymaking throughout the province.
As of 2018, public health sector unions have not ratified collective agreements that were negotiated under the new Health Authority Act in 2015.

8.2 Equity in financing the health care system

Nova Scotia's top corporate tax rate, at 16 per cent, is (along with that of
Prince Edward Island) the highest in Canada. Its small-business tax rate,
at 3 per cent, is close to the national average. Despite the high tax rate
for corporations, however, a relatively small percentage of total income
tax is derived from corporate income tax. Of total tax revenue for 2015,
54.3 per cent was from income tax (personal and corporate), while 42.6
per cent came from consumption taxes. Of the $2,783,967 gathered in
total income tax, 84.1 per cent was from personal income tax, and 15.9
per cent was derived from corporate taxes. Of total provincial tax revenue (income plus consumption), then, only about 8 per cent is provided
through a tax on corporations (Nova Scotia, 2015c). This breakdown of
tax revenue reflects the structural limitations noted in chapter 1: the
province depends on a very small number of very large corporations to

Figure 8.1 Sources of total provincial tax revenue, Nova Scotia, 2015

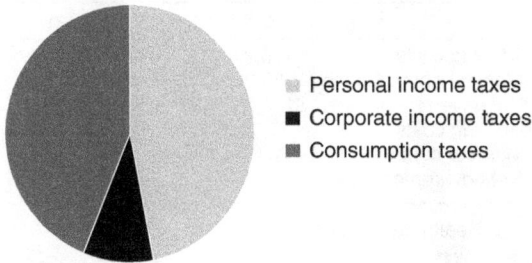

- Personal income taxes
- Corporate income taxes
- Consumption taxes

Source: *Nova Scotia: Public Accounts 2015*, vol. 1, p. 48. Available at http://www
.novascotia.ca/finance/en/home/publications/publicaccounts.aspx

employ Nova Scotians. A large number of very small businesses provide only a very small proportion of employment positions and tax revenue. Consequently, the province focuses on attracting and retaining large corporate enterprises through large subsidies. Notwithstanding the high formal tax rate for large corporations, mechanisms such as payroll rebates are employed to offset these higher rates. Between 2004–5 and 2014–15, the province granted over $88 million in payroll rebates (Nova Scotia Business Inc., personal communication, 15 March 2016). In November 2014, the new Liberal government released a review of Nova Scotia's tax system. The Broten report suggested eliminating exemptions for sales taxes on items such as books, children's clothing, shoes, diapers, feminine hygiene products, and residential fuel costs; removing the top tax bracket on those earning more than $150,000 per year; and lowering the top corporate tax rate from 16 per cent to 13.5 per cent (Broten, 2014). None of these recommendations were enacted. As Figure 8.1 illustrates, and as noted above, the vast majority of public funding for provincial expenditure comes from personal income tax (45.7 per cent) and consumption taxes (42.6 per cent); only 8.6 per cent of total tax revenue in Nova Scotia is obtained from corporate taxes (Nova Scotia, 2015c).

The discussion over who ought to bear health-related costs was brought into stark relief in 2016, when the DHW attempted to shift the costs of the Seniors' Pharmacare program towards the recipients through the restructuring of premiums. Unlike the province's other pharmacare programs, the Seniors' Pharmacare program had not been a means-tested program, but one based purely on age. All seniors who opted into the voluntary program paid the same premiums. The Seniors' Pharmacare

Table 8.1 Nova Scotia Seniors' Pharmacare cost sources, 5-year projection

		2015–16	2020–1
Before policy change	Total drug costs	$166,210,000	$216,202,247
	Member contributions	$53,000,000	$67,044,349
	Net government cost	$113,210,000	$149,157,898
Projection assuming all	Total drug costs		$216,202,247
beneficiaries stay in the	Member contributions		$71,299,513
program	Net government cost		$144,902,734

Source: Nova Scotia Department of Health and Wellness, 2016.

Program Regulations (supporting the Fair Drug Pricing Act) had for years specified that the cost-sharing of the Seniors' Pharmacare program would be held at a constant ratio of 75 per cent from government funds to 25 per cent from individuals' premiums. This stipulation of a 75:25 ratio was quietly repealed by the government through orders in council in January 2015. A year later, a means-tested reform of the Seniors' Pharmacare program was announced. A press release from the DHW declared that "12,000 seniors who previously paid a premium won't pay one this year," although it failed to note that other seniors would be paying much more than they previously had (Nova Scotia Department of Health and Wellness, 2016b). The press release also did not mention that within five years, 33 per cent of the program's costs (up from 25 per cent) would come from premiums (Table 8.1). After a public outcry, the province backed down from its plan to increase premiums for the Seniors' Pharmacare program and stated that no further changes would be made until seniors' groups had been consulted.

8.3 Equity of access

As previous chapters have documented, the issue of geographical equity of access to health care services underlies much policy discussion in Nova Scotia. To an extent, it informed the decision to consolidate the DHAs in 2015. As in most Canadian provinces, the problem of providing equitable services in a population characterized by increasing urbanization and growing rural depopulation is difficult and complex. As the DHW's 2015–16 Statement of Mandate acknowledges, "there continue to be distribution challenges affecting equitable access for all Nova Scotians, especially in rural communities" (2015d, 6). These challenges have many causes, including the need to achieve scale economies when providing many health care services, and the difficulty of attracting health care professionals to remote areas. Rural inhabitants will never enjoy the same level of many services, such as specialized and tertiary ones, and the determination of what "equitable" means given physical and economic limitations is a highly political issue.

Income is also a variable that influences equity of access. As Asada and Kephart (2007) and Hajizadeh (2017) have pointed out, socioeconomic inequities have an impact on access to health care services across Canada notwithstanding the existence of universal health insurance. Socioeconomic status also influences the type of health care services accessed. Kephart, Thomas, and Maclean (1998) found that the use of physician services in Nova Scotia was inversely associated with socioeconomic status. Allin (2008) has corroborated this data and added that those with higher incomes in Nova Scotia were more likely to access specialist care, while those with lower incomes tended to use more hospital care. These trends were similar across most Canadian provinces.

Other factors that may impede access to health services include ethnicity, gender, and sexual orientation. The extent of such barriers to access has not been extensively quantified, although there is anecdotal evidence of inequity in access to health care services in the province (Sharif, Dar, & Amaratunga, 2000). The former Capital Health District Authority was quite engaged in developing a diversity and inclusion strategy. A Diversity and Inclusion Steering Committee was formed in 2003 to support efforts by First Nations, African Nova Scotians, immigrants, and francophones to access appropriate care, and 2 years later expanded to include other marginalized groups. In 2007, a full-time diversity and inclusion coordinator was hired by Capital Health, and in 2010 the health authority completed its first workforce diversity survey. The DHW has also issued general "cultural competence" guidelines.

8.4 Outcomes

8.4.1 Comparative outcomes

Notwithstanding the poor health indicators that characterize Nova Scotia, the key outcomes for health system performance in the province are reasonably good. As chapter 1 noted, Nova Scotians tend to be more overweight than Canadians on average; have higher rates of cancer, diabetes, high blood pressure, arthritis, heart disease, and respiratory disease than the rest of Canada; and consume fewer fruits and vegetables

Table 8.2 Health system performance indicators, Nova Scotia and Canada, 2013

Outcome Measure	Metric	Nova Scotia	Canada
Accessibility	Influenza immunization less than one year ago, %	44.5	29.3
	Has a regular medical doctor, %	90.3	84.5
Appropriateness	Caesarean section, %	27.1	27.3
	Patients with repeat hospitalizations for mental illness, % (2012 data)	10.5	11.0
Continuity	30-day readmission rate for mental illness, %	11.1	11.5
Effectiveness	30-day acute myocardial infarction readmission, %	9.2	11.4
	30-day medical readmission, %	12.8	13.5
Safety	Hospitalized hip-fracture event rate, age standardized, per 100,000	505	445

Sources: Statistics Canada, CANSIM Table 105–0501; CIHI Health System Performance Indicators http://www.cihiconferences.ca/indicators/2015/tables15_e.html

but more alcohol and tobacco. Nonetheless, the province does perform very close to the national average on key health system performance indicators established by the Canadian Institute for Health Information (CIHI) (Table 8.2). On the measurement of "accessibility," for example, where 2013 data is available, Nova Scotia scores better than the national average on two indicators (influenza immunization and access to a regular medical doctor) and worse on one (wait time for hip-fracture surgery). On the evaluation of "appropriateness," the province is marginally better on both indicators (C-sections and patients with repeat hospitalizations for mental illness). Nova Scotia's measurement on "continuity" (30-day readmission rate for mental illness) is also slightly better than the national average. For two main indicators for "effectiveness," Nova Scotia performs slightly better (30-day acute myocardial readmission and 30-day medical readmission), although the province scores worse for the single "safety" indicator (hospitalized hip-fracture event rate).

8.4.2 Chronological outcomes

In addition to evaluating outcomes with reference to other jurisdictions, one can assess outcomes by examining trends over time within a single jurisdiction. The DHW's annual accountability reports attempt to address the question of how well the provincial system has been performing over time. The performance measures employed in the 2013–14 and 2014–15 reports focus on wait times for mental health services; utilization rates and wait times for emergency services; use of electronic health records; and rates of nutrition, smoking, and alcohol consumption (the measurement of gambling rates was discontinued after 2013–14).

The figures for emergency services are a particularly interesting set of indicators, as they address the period of policy reform for emergency health care that began in 2010. On the one hand, the rate of individuals waiting within the benchmark period has remained almost unchanged between 2011 and 2015 (between 86 to 87 per cent of patients with serious conditions were seen within eight hours, with a goal benchmark of 90 per cent). But the number of individuals presenting in emergency departments for minor conditions has dropped from 57 to 50 per cent over the same period, which would seem to indicate that certain aspects of the emergency care redesign (such as utilization of collaborative emergency centres or the practice of elderly patients in long-term care being attended by paramedics on-site) may be working well. This figure is even more remarkable when juxtaposed with figures showing an *increase* in unscheduled closure times for CECs between 2012 and 2015 from 0.7 per cent to 1.6 per cent closure of scheduled hours (Nova Scotia Department of Health and Wellness, 2015e).

Another success is reflected in breastfeeding rates: both the percentage of infants who have received early breast contact (72.7 per cent in 2006 to 85.0 per cent in 2013), and the percentage of infants who exclusively breastfed for at least six months (18.8 per cent in 2005 to 31.9 per cent in 2013–14), have significantly increased. Another notable point is the increase in access to electronic health records. From 2011 to 12 to 2014–15, the total number of clinical users of the Secure Health Access Record (SHARE) climbed from 475 to 4,858, a tenfold increase. Technically, this figure is a surrogate endpoint, as it is not a direct indicator of health. Rather, it implies a correlation between the utilization of electronic health records and improvement of health outcomes. The data only stated the numbers of clinicians using SHARE, and did not indicate the percentage of clinicians doing so.

Nova Scotia performed much more poorly on indicators for nutrition, smoking, and alcohol consumption. The percentage of Nova Scotians consuming at least five servings of fruits and vegetables daily fell from a high of 38.3 per cent in 2009 to a low of 30.9 per cent in 2014; and the percentage of those over the age of 25 who smoked actually increased from 15.6 per cent in 2012 to 19.4 per cent in 2013. Similarly, the percentage of Nova Scotians drinking in excess has increased from 2011 to 2013. One must interpret these statistics with caution. It may possibly be the case that more Nova Scotians are engaging in poor lifestyle choices. However, it may also be the case that individual behaviour per se is not changing, and that the significant exodus of younger, healthier adults seeking employment outside the province reflects a higher proportion of those (possibly in higher age ranges or in poorer health) who remain in the province. Nova Scotia has in recent years focused on smoking prevention among youths (including a ban on both the sale of flavoured tobacco and on the sale of e-cigarettes to minors), and it is worth noting that the rates of smoking for those between the ages of 15 and 19 have decreased from 16 per cent in 2010 to 10 per cent in 2013.

Mental health outcomes are much more ambivalent. Access to mental health services has been an important political issue, especially for youth, and the province has been attempting to address these problems. But it is difficult to evaluate the outcomes. Data shows that the percentages of child and adolescent clients seen in urgent cases (within 7 days) and in regular cases (within 90 days) have both improved. However, the percentage of these individuals seen in semi-urgent cases (within 30 days) has dropped precipitously. In 2010–11, for example, 57 per cent of urgent cases, 51 per cent of semi-urgent cases, and 70 per cent of urgent cases met the standard, but in 2013–14, 56 per cent of urgent cases, 15 per cent of semi-urgent, and 89 per cent of regular cases met their respective standards (Nova Scotia Department of Health and Wellness, 2014): because the measurement of wait times for mental health services changed midway through the 2014–15 reporting period, no data on mental health wait times were presented in the 2014–15 accountability report.

Overall, these outcome measures are not entirely unproblematic. There is, for example, no clear explanation of why certain indicators were chosen rather than others; nor are the outcomes to be measured explicitly stated in advance of the evaluation process. Just as measurable outcomes must be stated before clinical trials commence, so too should policy outcomes (along with the metrics being used to assess these outcomes) be publicly articulated before analysis of the data begins to avoid cherry-picking positive indicators. There is putative progress in the area of performance evaluation; both the DHW's Statement of Mandate for 2014–2015 and its *Accountability Report: 2015–2016* stated that the department was in the process of designing an accountability framework that would measure the system's performance in relation to health of the population, experience of care, health system workforce, and resource stewardship. Under this framework, key performance indicators, first-year goals, and outcome-based targets would be articulated. However, if these indicators do exist, they are not yet accessible to the general public. The DHW's *Accountability Report: 2016–2017*, for example, is simply a list of current and planned projects. An appendix provides only five carefully curated "performance highlights" based on minimal data. For an "accountability report" to be of any real use, it must select indicators well in advance (so that outcomes are not selectively chosen); indicators must be comprehensive; the same indicators must be used from year to year so that it is possible to gauge progress; and these data must be accessible to the public. The DHW's accountability reports fail on all of these fronts.

8.4.3 Measuring and evaluating outcomes

Separate from the discussion of actual health outcomes, but highly relevant to it, is the consideration of the capacity of the province effectively to evaluate outcomes. To determine the evaluative capacity of a province, one must ask whether data is collected; whether the data can be effectively juxtaposed to proper comparators; and whether the information can be easily accessed and used by those who need it. The biggest obstacle to the development of a strong capacity to evaluate outcomes is the fragmentation of information, although this fragmentation occurs in a number of different ways.

The most obvious example of fragmentation is geographical. When discrete DHAs within the former regionalized system had much responsibility to compile data, there was often little explicit standardization of the way in which information was presented. While the Capital District Health Authority (CDHA) measured wait times for mental health services using the median and 90th percentile, for example, other DHAs tracked wait times according to urgent, semi-urgent, and regular priority standards. Following consolidation, all zones will be reporting wait-times data in a more consistent manner. Similarly, electronic health records were still not fully interoperational in 2017; a physician in an emergency department in Dartmouth, for example, could not electronically access a child's medical records at the IWK Health Centre.

Another problem is that even where consistent endpoint data exists, it is not necessarily tied to program evaluation. For example, each 811 telephone call that provides immediate access to a nurse is considerably more costly than a general GP visit. However, its value could be defended on the grounds that it provides access to medical advice after hours, when most GPs are unavailable, and access to medical advice for those who are geographically isolated. At the same, time, however, the 811 service was experiencing "lower than anticipated call volumes" by 2014–15. So is the 811 service good value for money, all things considered? No one knows, as the program has not been evaluated.

Another form of fragmentation rests in the lack of accessibility to data. There are four main administrative health databases in Nova Scotia (vital statistics, discharge abstracts, drug claims, and physician claims), which can be accessed via Health Data Nova Scotia. However, much of this information exists in the form of scanned PDFs and so cannot be easily sorted or aggregated. There are also nine clinical databases that correspond to specific conditions (e.g., heart disease, cancer, diabetes, depression, reproductive care), as well as a separate diagnostic database (which includes information systems such as PACS). Complicated linkage processes are required to use this information effectively in order to measure and evaluate how well particular aspects of the health system are operating, but as these databases must all be accessed separately, such linkages are extremely difficult to construct. Interpreting the data within these databases is also a problem, as there is no standardized approach to very basic issues such as case definition (i.e., how a condition is defined). Thus, independent researchers using the same database but different methods to define conditions may well produce data that is conflicting or difficult to compare.

The evaluation of outcomes and the development of new policy is also hampered by the lack of capacity. Formally, "policy capacity" refers not only to the bank of technical skills and disciplinary knowledge that a government can call on but also to a pool of understanding of the feasibility and strategies of implementing and nurturing policies after the design stage (Denis et al., 2015). Smaller jurisdictions tend, unsurprisingly, to have less policy capacity in many respects: they can afford to hire only a small number of policy analysts, and those they have tend to spend more time addressing short-term "brushfires" than long-term planning. But even compared to smaller provinces such as Manitoba or Saskatchewan, Nova Scotia has very limited capacity for policy evaluation. There is, for example, no arms-length health-policy institute to provide objective assessments of how well policies and programs work, or to design new policies and programs. This puts the province at a considerable disadvantage in evaluative capacity compared to a province like Ontario, which established the Institute for Clinical Evaluative Sciences (ICES) in

1992. ICES administers seven separate research programs (one of which is health system planning and evaluation) and has access to numerous linked data sets (e.g., from the Cardiac Care Network of Ontario and Cancer Care Ontario, as well as from individual hospitals, laboratories, pharmacies, and long-term care facilities), which are overseen by expert teams of data-quality and data-management specialists (Dolan et al., 2012). It secures consistent and predictable funding from the government of Ontario and, at a rate of $0.80 per resident of Ontario, it has an operating budget of more than 10 million dollars per year. In addition to ICES, Ontario utilizes information produced by Health Quality Ontario, which focuses on performance evaluation and quality improvement. In comparison, Nova Scotia's Health Data NS unit is funded on a limited and ad hoc basis, with a very minimal support staff.

In sum, the overarching problem is that poor evaluative capacity gives rise to a vicious circle: spending money on programs and policies that do not work well means that demand for health services is not effectively addressed; channeling more resources into meeting this demand in turn means that there are fewer resources to be employed in assessing how well existing programs function. The problem, according to some, is exacerbated by the trend to "new public governance," in which various accountability regimes are imposed on governments, in addition to the rise of social media, which has made governments shift into a mode of "court government." This is a model in which decisions are increasingly made at the centre, and polices are increasingly made by political staff (with no technical expertise) rather than by career civil servants (Savoie, 2015). Without a solid base for policy evaluation and outcomes assessment, there is little balance to policy design driven more by politics than by evidence.

8.4.4 User experience and satisfaction

The reporting of patient experiences in Nova Scotia is also fragmented. There have been two axes of fragmentation: by DHA and by program. Until 2015, authority to collect patient data rested with individual DHAs. The CDHA, for example, had collected and published user experience data through its Patient Experience Reporting System (PERS) since 2011. Patient experience data from other DHAs is very difficult to find. The CDHA used random samples of inpatient, ambulatory, and rehabilitation patients. In the 2013–14 fiscal year, the survey collected 3,801 responses (a response rate of 33.3 per cent). This survey (see Table 8.3)

Table 8.3 Patient Experience Survey Results Summary, April 2013–March 2014

Capital Health – Inpatient

Answer group	Overall assessment of care received	Emergency department	Continuity and coordination of care	Care received from health professional	Respect for rights	Concern for safely	Facility environment	All surveys
Positive	90%	89%	84%	91%	92%	78%	77%	87%
Negative	10%	11%	16%	9%	8%	22%	23%	13%

Capital Health – Ambulatory Care

Answer group	Overall assessment of care received	Accessibility of services	Continuity and coordination of care	Care received from health professional	Respect for rights	Concern for safely	Facility environment	All surveys
Positive	94%	91%	89%	96%	94%	93%	91%	93%
Negative	6%	9%	11%	4%	6%	7%	9%	7%

Source: CDHA, Patient Experience Survey Results, https://www.cdha.nshealth.ca/about-us/measuring-success-progress/patient-experience-survey

Table 8.4 Patient satisfaction with health care services received in the past 12 months, 2005

	Nova Scotia	Canada
Very or somewhat satisfied with health care services received, %	89.2	85.0
Very or somewhat satisfied with family doctor or other physician care received, %	94.5	91.3
Very or somewhat satisfied with community-based health care, %	86.3	82.0

Source: CANSIM Table 105–0280, http://www5.statcan.gc.ca/cansim/a26?lang=eng&id=1050083.

simply asked respondents to rate their experiences as "positive" or "negative," with a satisfactory response rate set at 90 per cent.

This information is difficult to compare with other provinces, as data from Statistics Canada go up only to 2005. According to these data, however, Nova Scotia compares quite favourably to the Canadian average (Table 8.4).

While some patient satisfaction data was collected on a geographical basis, other information has been captured by specific programs (as noted in chapter 8, section 4.3). Information on patient experiences with cancer care in Nova Scotia, for example, was collected in patient surveys conducted in 2007, 2009, and 2011. Again, patient satisfaction in the most recent survey remains comparable to, or above, the national average in all metrics (Canadian Partnership against Cancer, 2016). In 2017, the NSHA released the first patient experience survey under the aegis of the new province-wide health authority, with an overall satisfaction rate of 89.5 per cent.

8.5 Efficiency

The evaluation of efficiency in the provision of health care services is a complex and difficult task. The rhetoric of allocative efficiency – and especially transferring resources from administrative tasks to "front line" services – played a large role in the most recent set of health care reforms. Yet there is little sound appraisal of this approach: the CIHI, for example, reports that administrative costs declined from 4.8 per cent in 2011–12 to 4.5 per cent in 2013–14 (*before* the current reforms were implemented), and that Nova Scotia's administrative expenses in health care are now on par with the Canadian average (CIHI, n.d., administrative expense details). Part of the problem with discussions of efficiency is the complex and interdependent nature of modern health care systems. Often a practice meant to increase the efficient utilization of resources in the short term can lead to long-term inefficiencies: hospitals like the Victoria General, for example, have become able to allocate hospital beds more efficiently; but running all wards at full capacity 24 hours a day for 12 months of the year means that there is no longer any opportunity to perform thorough maintenance on closed wards (Nova Scotia Office of the Auditor General, 2016b, 34). Consequently, the physical integrity of hospitals wards is now deteriorating at a much faster pace.

Occasionally, maximizing efficient practices in one unit will lead to inefficient practices in another. To keep the repair costs down, a diagnostic unit may choose to wait until regular business hours to have important equipment repaired; but if emergency departments do not have access to these diagnostic services over nights or weekends, they will have to use ambulances to take patients to other hospitals for diagnostic services, thus driving up overall costs and as well as inconvenience to patients. Another problem is balancing technical efficiency with other values, such as perceived quality. This is the issue underlying the political controversy over home-care reform: a formal tendered service contract could mean that more cost savings might be achieved; but those receiving (and providing) these services have expressed a concern that this shift would mean a diminution in the quality of care they currently receive from providers that they know. It is also potentially disquieting that the province posted a savings of $2.2 million in public health due to lower utilization rates for vaccination programs and lower spending in chronic-disease and injury-prevention initiatives (Nova Scotia Department of Health and Wellness, 2015e), $28 million due to delays on major construction projects, and $6 million due to delays in IT projects (Nova Scotia Department of Health and Wellness, 2016c). Depending on the specific nature of these reduced utilizations or program delays, it is possible that lower spending in these areas may ultimately mean higher spending in acute, long-term, or other areas in the future.

Part of the problem, as noted above, is that the province does not necessarily have the capacity to determine whether its spending patterns are efficient or not. For example, in 2014–15 the province spent $3.6 million in insured services to finance an increasing number of visits by Nova Scotians for hospital services in other provinces. This spending could be efficient or inefficient, depending on the relative cost of providing the services locally (is there a critical mass of patients who require one kind of treatment for which the province might usefully develop a local treatment base?), but detailed information on this kind of spending must be available to make this determination. Nova Scotia's health reforms have included a commitment to introduce systematic approaches to the efficient utilization of health care resources. A health services plan is being created and "will serve as the foundation for many decisions in the health system" to improve "patient outcomes and effective and efficient use of system resources" (Nova Scotia Department of Health and Wellness, 2015e, 8). A collaborative care framework is being developed in order that the scopes of practice for all health care professionals are being used most effectively. Also, a One Person, One Record health information system is being pursued in order to achieve "a single person-centric information system that will provide a more cohesive and cost-effective operational environment" (ibid., 9). Yet each of these systems is still under some level of development, and it is still too early to evaluate their utility.

8.6 Transparency and accountability

There is no formal health technology assessment unit in Nova Scotia. Unlike many other provinces, Nova Scotia depends solely on pan-Canadian agencies and processes such as the Common Drug Review. It is thus difficult to know why particular kinds of health technologies are, or are not, funded by the province. Generally, in making such a determination, the DHW will consult with experts in the field when considering whether to use particular devices, procedures, or drugs. The assumption, of course, is that both the province and health care professionals are making decisions based only on good evidence and best practices. Yet there is no way of knowing whether or not this is the case with each particular decision. Governments in general can and have made policy decisions based on poor evidence to appease particular constituencies. In 2010, for example, four provinces agreed to conduct clinical trials for Paolo Zamboni's "liberation therapy" treatment for multiple sclerosis in the face of political pressure from patient advocacy groups. (Nova Scotia's health minister refused to dedicate resources to clinical trials on the grounds that there was insufficient evidence to support such an allocation.) By 2014, these clinical trials had confirmed that the treatment was indeed ineffective (Traboulsee et al., 2014). Likewise, the practice of consulting informally with disciplinary experts can be problematic given that such individuals may show a preference for treatments or technologies with which they are involved. There is no evidence to show that this is occurring, but the lack of transparency in such decision-making practices also means that there is no evidence that it does not happen.

Accountability is a slightly more complex concept. In health systems there are at least two discrete modes of accountability. One addresses oversight of, and responsibility for, decisions that result in negative outcomes. Prior to the 2015–16 reforms, the oversight for quality and safety issues rested in the DHW. In 2016, the oversight function was passed to the newly created NSHA. While quality and safety issues in DHAs were overseen by the DHW under the former system, they are now the provenance of the NSHA, leading some to worry that the concept of self-policing is neither an effective nor appropriate principle of governance for a health system. The DHW has responded that it will remain ultimately responsible for oversight on quality and safety issues; but this leads to an administrative tension. On the one hand, if oversight remains at the level of the NSHA, the province will simply not know whether there is in fact an issue of concern unless it is flagged for their attention. On the other hand, if the DHW becomes too involved in the minutiae of oversight, it will compromise the clear distinction between "policy formation" and "management" on which the reorganization of the health system was based.

A second mode of accountability focusses on whether or not those at the helm of a health system have met the benchmarks and other outcome measures against which the performance of the health system is to be measured. The DHW publishes annual accountability reports but, as noted above, it is not clear why particular indicators (or targets) were chosen rather than others. Moreover, while each year's accountability report outlines "where we are now?" and "where do we want to be in the future?" for each category, the previous year's targets are not mentioned, so one does not know the extent to which the previous year's objectives were met unless one refers directly to the previous year's reports. Even then, this data may not be included, as the indicators chosen for inclusion in the accountability reports vary considerably from year to year. Some of the declared outcomes are also quite vague: the 2013–14 report, for example, presents very nonspecific benchmarks ("DHW wants to see a downward trend in the percentage of CTAS 4-5 patients being seen in the emergency department") or aspirational statements in place of quantifiable metrics, as it does in other categories ("Our goal is to provide predictable and sustainable access to health care in Nova Scotia and to minimize unscheduled closures in these communities"). The 2015–16 DHW Statement of Mandate and the 2015–16 NSHA Business Plan state that performance measures are being developed. In 2015–16, according to its Statement of Mandate, the DHW "will be implementing an accountability framework to better articulate what it expects from the Nova Scotia Health Authority and IWK Health Centre" (13). The 2015–16 NSHA Business Plan outlines 21 indicators in this new accountability framework and notes that specific targets to be provided and approved by the DHW are "currently under development" (11). Comprehensive outcomes established by this accountability framework were not included in the 2016–17 accountability report. However, by 2017 the NSHA created a website that listed a comprehensive set of key indicators for 2016–17.

8.7 Summary

Given the scope and newness of Nova Scotia's health reforms, it is difficult to make a detailed assessment of the current system at this point. Politically, one of the key stated objectives of the reforms – overall administrative efficiency leading to cost savings – will take time properly to evaluate. On the one hand, the NSHA's ability to procure and to allocate goods and services on a province-wide basis would seem to be a useful step towards this goal; on the other hand, the province's focus on annual balanced-budget financing may have a detrimental long-term impact on infrastructure. The health care reforms have also taken precedence for several years over the development of long-term strategic planning in areas such as primary care, continuing care, and mental health care, all of which are still in preparation. Collaborative care is seen as the broad foundation for such programmatic shifts, but the lack of clarity regarding the role and oversight of physicians and physician services presents a major organizational hurdle to this end. Progress in health IT, and especially in the development of the province-wide MyHealthNS personal health record system, is a promising event; but, again, the implementation of this system depends on ongoing discussions with physicians regarding payment options.

In terms of health human performance, Nova Scotia has built up a much more detailed bank of knowledge regarding the province's health care professionals and has complemented this with a needs-based plan for health care workers into the future. However, the overall economic situation in the province means that professional remuneration is rarely competitive nationally, and relations between the government and the public sector unions are brittle and acrimonious. The new reforms, which have centralized most services and programs within a single health authority, depend on a zonal structure to address regional representation. Whether, and how well, the new system can accommodate both the efficiencies of centralization and responsiveness to local concerns remains to be determined. Notwithstanding all these underlying issues, health care outcomes based on select national indicators are reasonably good in Nova Scotia compared to other provinces. However, given the proportion of public spending directed to health care, and given changes to the way in which federal funds are calculated, there is real concern regarding the sustainability of this level of performance.

Chapter Nine

Conclusion

Health care in Canada, writ large, is the combined narrative of decisions and strategies undertaken by individual provinces and territories (Lazar, Lavis, Forest, & Church, 2013). The decentralization of health care is perhaps more pronounced in Canada than in any other developed nation (Requejo, 2010), and the need to understand the granularity of experience is consequently important in Canadian health systems research. Because of the complexity and expense of contemporary health care, observes Greer (forthcoming), relatively small variations in outcomes across regional jurisdictions "can have interesting politics and big consequences." The fiscal capacity, political culture, institutional framework, and leadership of each province and territory have a strong influence on the way in which health care is provided. At the same time, however, it is easy to become so immersed in the granularity of provincial systems that one loses sight of the larger context within which provincial policymaking takes place. As the relationship between Ottawa and the provinces deteriorated under the Harper administration, so the horizontal relationships between provinces began to take on more importance. This, coupled with an incoming federal administration in 2015 pursuing a more engaged social infrastructure agenda, means that provinces may have more capacity-building opportunities in health care that extend beyond provincial boundaries. International variables are also important to consider: financial trends can have sudden and forceful impacts on the capability of provinces to offer new programs or pay for existing ones; and intellectual fashions in organizational theory can have a considerable, if more gradual, effect on the way in which decision makers choose to organize structures of health system funding, delivery, and governance (Koon, Hawkins & Mayhew 2016).

If a broader focus makes us aware of how little room any province has for substantial policy change, a narrower focus nonetheless allows us to see the enormous complexity and difficulty involved even in maintaining what already exists. As a former Nova Scotia cabinet minister wryly observed,

> It is beyond the capacity of any single person to exert meaningful control over such a complex system. It would make more sense for half the cabinet to be health ministers. One of them could be the senior minister, and the others could be associate ministers responsible for the other big pieces of the health-care puzzle: people, infrastructure, quality, long-term care, acute care, and pharmacare. At least that would make more sense than the current system, where we have one health minister who can barely hang on, sitting around the table with a bunch of mini-ministers who are responsible for not very much at all. (Steele, 2016)

As modern health care becomes more intricate – more a series of reticulated systems than a single structure – the need to address governance in a logical and disciplined manner has become more pressing. In Nova Scotia, as in most other provinces (and many states worldwide), the attempt to reconfigure governance structures to address this complexity has been expressed through the meme of regionalization. The notable health care reforms in Nova Scotia have been efforts to establish regionalized structures (1994), to deepen regionalization (2001), and to reduce regionalization (2015). In each case the attempt was not so much to disperse or consolidate authority as it was more clearly to clarify the division of responsibilities between those designing policy (steering) and those delivering services (rowing). Given the province's experimentation over two decades with several different types of regionalization, then, it is remarkable that so many issues have remained constant over time: concerns over long-term care and chronic illness, for example, were articulated in reports going back to 1950.

There are at least two reasons for this obdurate lack of any real progress in addressing these concerns though strategies of regionalization. One is the presumption that the relevant decisions are the ones made at the top, rather than those made at the point of patient contact. A health care system is, to a large extent, merely the concatenation of small decisions made every day by those within the system. By drawing an emphatic artificial line between those who "make" and those who "execute" policy, it is possible to lose sight of the need to understand why these small but important decisions are made in the first place. This was originally the profound insight of "patient centred care," although the term has become often little more than a hollow rhetorical flourish decorating policy directives.

A second reason for the limited success of regionalization is that the expected outcomes of the strategy have been remarkably inchoate over the years. The rhetoric of both more and less regionalization has, in Nova Scotia, always included references to efficiency and fairness. But both efficiency and fairness are slippery terms. The original premise of New Public Management was that centralized control was a cumbersome and inefficient form of organizing health systems because the decision makers at the top were too distant from service provision to know exactly what resources and strategies were required to treat specific patients in specific places. Giving those who had a better sense of local need more control over decision making at the municipal or regional level meant greater allocative efficiency. The poor responsiveness of centralized decision making was a clear theme, for example, in the 1989 Gallant report, which argued that more regionalization in health system governance would "result in effective and efficient use of existing capital" (15). The 2015 reforms in contrast, focused on the inefficiencies inherent in the intrinsic fragmentation of a regionalized system, and addressed the gains to technical efficiency arising from the scale economies inherent in a consolidated system.

Likewise, both the shift to regionalization undertaken in 1994 and 2001, and the move away from it in 2015, were articulated within a discourse of democratic legitimacy. The original model of regionalization in Nova Scotia, as chapter 2 describes, was to be one in which both citizens (through community health boards) and providers (through devolved management structures) had the opportunity to become more engaged. In contrast, the consolidation of DHAs in 2015 was justified with reference to its capacity to provide "greater equity" to health care users across all regions. "Regionalization," as a strategy, cannot by itself provide simple solutions to the complex problems facing modern health care systems because the concept contains ambiguous meanings and irreconcilable tensions (Marchildon, 2016). If real decision-making power is devolved downwards because it is important to respond to local concerns, some fragmentation must occur. And if services are amalgamated to establish scale economies in the equitable provision of services across all regions, then opportunities for real decision making at a local level will be curtailed. If we do not identify exactly what it is that we desire from a strategy of regionalization, and if we refuse to acknowledge what is lost as well as what is gained from such a process, it is hardly surprising that we find it difficult to evaluate the outcomes of regionalization despite the length and breadth of experience we have had with it.

Nova Scotia's health care system faces some daunting challenges. The demand for services is, and will continue to be, exacerbated by a higher proportion of older adults and higher rates of chronic disease in the province. Depopulation in many areas of the province decreases the cost-effectiveness with which traditional health care services can be offered in rural areas. And given that that health care accounts for almost half of provincial spending, Nova Scotia's financial circumstances will continue to have a substantial impact on the long-term sustainability of the province's health care system. Nonetheless, one must be careful how one interprets the relationship between the province's economy and the health care sector. Given the relative size of the province's economy, and the high proportion of public funds consumed by health care, it is not surprising to see that Nova Scotia performs worse than all provinces excepting only Prince Edward Island and New Brunswick in terms of program expenses relative to GDP. When measured according to program expenses per capita, however, Nova Scotia actually spends less than all provinces except for Ontario, Quebec, and British Columbia (RBC, 2016). Moreover, while the province is struggling with its debt load, its net debt to GDP ratio, as well as its net debt per capita, are both much sounder than those of either Ontario or Quebec (ibid.). In sum, while economic conditions pose serious challenges to the ongoing sustainability of Nova Scotia's health care system, the province is by no means an outlier compared to other Canadian provinces.

When considering health outcomes relative to other provinces, too, Nova Scotia is able to provide reasonable services notwithstanding its smaller size and limited economic base, although wait times are generally longer. Health care programs are a priority for the province. Nova Scotians expect to receive a certain level of services within a particular period of time; and the province is generally quite responsive to public demands regarding the provision of specific services. Moreover, sufficient benchmarks exist to be able to compare the performance of provinces across Canada in providing health care services, which imposes a certain amount of political pressure on each province not to fall too far behind the others. More problematic, however, is the sustainability of the province's capital infrastructure. Unlike the services provided to patients at point of contact, the physical infrastructure of the province's health care system is generally not quite as visible to the general public. When there are serious constraints on provincial health care funding, the burden will be borne by "invisible" aspects of the health care system that are ignored by the public, and by long-term spending programs that carry no short-term political advantages. Capital infrastructure falls into both of these categories. The facilities and equipment on which health care in Nova Scotia depends is severely compromised, and there is little political will to address the problem (through comprehensive upkeep or replacement) until it clearly becomes a political crisis. Unlike services, it is difficult to evaluate the relative state of a province's infrastructure relative to other jurisdictions on an ongoing basis. Health care providers working in and with this infrastructure are those who are most likely to apprehend the deficiencies in the physical plant; yet at the same time they cannot be unaware that public funds marked for wages and salaries compete with funding for upkeep and renewal. For any government attempting to balance the provision of health care services, the refurbishment of health infrastructure, and a balanced health care budget, the path forward will be formidable.

A related deficiency is that of policy capacity. Policy capacity is the set of "intellectual and organizational resources" possessed by a government "that may be brought to bear on the policymaking process so as to design coherent, viable, and politically feasible policies" (Denis et al., 2015, 7). Policy capacity is an inchoate concept; but systems tend to work better when it flourishes and to struggle when it does not. While more nebulous a concept than physical infrastructure, policy capacity is another long-term investment required to facilitate the sustainability of health care systems over time. The complexity and technical detail of modern health care, the speed of change within the health care system, and the need for health systems iteratively to respond to changes mean that information, and the capacity to process information, have become just as important to sustainability as physical infrastructure.

One aspect of policy capacity is the ability to collect, interpret, and apply relevant information. Data must be collected at the granular level, but it must also be fed into information systems that permit the data to be compared and evaluated in an efficient and useful way. There must also be some policy development capability (either in-house or arms-length) that is able to translate this information into viable and effective policies. Policy development requires two quite separate kinds of skills. One is field-specific technical expertise: that is, the cadre of epidemiologists, economists, IT experts, lawyers, and experts in diseases, drugs, devices, and treatment protocols that is required to identify what is needed to address particular health issues. The other skill required is the ability to shepherd technical policies through the administrative and political landscape. Those who possess this ability are generally career civil servants with considerable experience. To the extent that these individuals are, as Savoie (2015) suggests, increasingly being marginalized by political staff who are more interested in designing politically attractive policies than sound administrative ones, a certain depth of judgment and understanding regarding what kinds of policies work and do not work is being lost.

A highly complex and technically specific health care system, then, requires an increasingly proficient administrative workforce able to collate, interpret, and evaluate the massive amounts of health data now available and to shape this information into evidence-based policies that are both technically appropriate and politically palatable. These skills and competencies are required regardless of the size of the jurisdiction: both smaller and larger provinces and territories will have the same range of medical conditions, treatments, policy options, and strategies to address. Larger jurisdictions, however, enjoy a critical mass and a taxation base that smaller ones do not. Thus, while health care may be improving considerably in an era increasingly informed by sophisticated technology and by the capacity to measure and evaluate treatments and policies, the ability for smaller jurisdictions to take advantage of this improvement is becoming severely compromised.

Nonetheless, small jurisdictional size can be a potential asset in health care policymaking. This is especially the case for Nova Scotia. As the province's health care system is designed to facilitate demand from all Atlantic provinces in specific areas, it has a greater technical capacity than a province of its size might otherwise exhibit. To this extent, it could potentially be able to "punch above its weight." The combination of sophisticated infrastructure and small scale does permit certain strategic advantages. One is the rather amorphous, although significant, existence of "social capital," including a greater personal familiarity among key decision makers that can precipitate a greater level of trust among stakeholders in smaller jurisdictions. An example of this is the development of the innovative Regulated Health Professions Network Act 2012, which permitted regulated health professionals to determine among themselves the way in which collaborative health care was to be developed. This kind of regulatory legislation evolved because of the small size of many of the self-regulated professions and because of the informal but intimate connections that already existed among the self-regulated professions. A related advantage of policymaking in smaller jurisdictions is the absence of multiple levels of bureaucratic formality in decision-making processes. Layers of formal accountability mechanisms and bureaucratic approval, especially concerning the approval of specific treatments and procedures, can delay and attenuate decision making in larger, more technocratic jurisdictions. Smaller jurisdictions can have more procedural flexibility. In 2009, for example, at the direct request of the minister and deputy minister of health, Nova Scotia fast-tracked the practice of giving tPA (a clot-busting stroke drug) to advanced paramedics.

Given the need for critical mass in developing and sustaining a sophisticated and technically complex health care system, smaller jurisdictions increasingly tend to be more willing to establish networks and collaborative enterprises that can provide a basis for scale economies. These undertakings can, in turn, lead to greater regional integration in a gradual and ad hoc manner. This integration is occurring both in the private and the public sector. Medavie EMS, for example, won the contract in 1998 for a province-wide system of emergency care to replace the fragmented private provision of ambulance services in the province. Since then it has built on its experience to develop ambulance services in New Brunswick, Prince Edward Island, and also small regions within Ontario and Massachusetts. The integration of public health services across the Atlantic provinces is also notable. New Brunswick, Prince Edward Island, and Newfoundland contract for services provided by the Queen Elizabeth II Health Sciences Centre and the IWK Children's Centre in Halifax. Dalhousie's School of Medicine holds seats for applicants from all three Maritime provinces and has established a regional campus in St. John for New Brunswick residents. In 2014, Nova Scotia and Prince Edward Island signed a joint agreement for 811 telehealth services. Therapeutic drugs for all four Atlantic provinces are evaluated by the Atlantic Common Drug Review. (Even after the establishment of the Common Drug Review in 2003, the Atlantic Common Drug Review still assesses some drugs that do not fall under the purview of the Common Drug Review.) Finally, the Atlantic Healthcare Collaboration for Innovation and Improvement in Chronic Disease, Quality Improvement Collaborative brings together health care organizations, health care providers, and patients across the Atlantic provinces (Rossiter et al., 2017).

Though based on necessity, Atlantic provinces nonetheless have experience in the integration and collaboration of health care services, and

Nova Scotia has often been the hub of this activity. It is arguable that effective health care is increasingly dependent on the ability to access larger data-driven systems, and that even larger jurisdictions will find an advantage in developing strategic alliances to identify best practices, streamline resources, and merge databases. The success of the pan-Canadian Pharmaceutical Alliance and the Canadian Partnership against Cancer are examples of the willingness of provinces both larger and smaller to collaborate to build a substantial capacity base that benefits all stakeholders. It is possible that Nova Scotia could use its experience in integration and collaboration across jurisdictions to help design a broader, more pan-Canadian health care framework that incorporates ground-up as well as top-down governance structures.

To date, however, the province lags behind many of the larger provinces in developing more systematic approaches in areas such as primary health care. The opportunities noted above are real; but taking advantage of them will require political leadership. The narrative of health reform in Nova Scotia is still being written, as it has for over two decades, in the language of regionalization. This is unfortunate, as no fixed point on the sliding scale from decentralization to consolidation will solve many of the underlying issues confronting the province's health care system. The demands of long-term and home care, the crumbling physical infrastructure, and the absence of coordinated data systems are all agnostic as to whether the geographical configuration of governance is centralized or decentralized. There are many advantages to consolidating service provision in health care: consistency in programs across regions, scale economies, mobility of personnel and equipment, better communication, IT compatibility, and coherent performance measures are better facilitated within a more centralized system (although this may, as noted earlier, come at the expense of ground-up engagement and responsiveness to local need). At the same time, however, the disruption occasioned by the substantial reform of the DHA structure and of the DHW itself means that deeper problems have not yet been addressed. The poor quality of health information has nothing to do with geographical regionalization per se; all of the fragmented databases are located within the Halifax Regional Municipality. The effort required to make this data serviceable is a political and administrative task independent of the specifics of governance structures. Likewise, the obvious need to restructure primary care to make it more accessible was not accomplished in the 2015–16 reforms.

It is difficult to evaluate systems while they are in the process of changing. Yet health care systems are rarely static. The technologies available to diagnose and treat illness, and to track and evaluate outcomes, have changed considerably in the past 25 years. Nonetheless, we are still thinking about the governance of health systems in terms of theories that became popular a quarter of a century ago. In the end, the deeper questions will increasingly be whether or not health systems can take advantage of such remarkable technological development, and how to do so in a way that addresses both the social values of the communities they serve and the political realities of democratic governance.

Appendix

Laws on Health and Health Care in Nova Scotia

- Anatomy Act
- Chiropractic Act
- Co-ordinated Home Care Act
- Counselling Therapists Act
- Dental Act
- Dental Hygienists Act
- Dental Technicians Act
- Denturists Act
- Doctors Nova Scotia Act
- Drug Dependency Foundation Act
- Emergency "911" Act
- Emergency Department Accountability Act
- Emergency Health Services Act
- Emergency Management Act
- Essential Health and Community Services Act
- Essential Home-support Services Act
- Fair Drug Pricing Act
- Health Act
- Health Authorities Act
- Health Council Act
- Health Council Appointments Act
- Health Protection Act
- Health Research Foundation Act
- Health Services and Insurance Act
- Healthcare Services Continuation Act
- Hospital Education Assistance Act
- Hospital Services Planning Commission Act

- Hospital Trusts Act
- Hospitals Act
- Human Organ and Tissue Donation Act (not proclaimed in force)
- Human Tissue Gift Act (repealed; repeal not proclaimed in force)
- Inebriates' Guardianship Act
- Involuntary Psychiatric Treatment Act
- Licensed Practical Nurses Act
- Long Term Disability Plan Ratification Act
- Medical Act
- Medical Imaging and Radiation Therapy Professionals Act (not proclaimed in force)
- Medical Laboratory Technology Act
- Medical Professional Corporations Act
- Medical Radiation Technologists Act
- Medical Services Act
- Midwifery Act
- Municipal Hospitals Loan Act
- Narcotic Drug Addicts Act
- Natural Products Act
- Naturopathic Doctors Act
- Nova Scotia Association of Health Organizations, An Act to Incorporate
- Nova Scotia Hospital Act
- Nova Scotia Sanatorium Act
- Occupational Health and Safety Act
- Occupational Therapists Act
- Optometry Act
- Paramedics Act
- Patient Safety Act
- Patients' Abandoned Property Act
- Personal Health Information Act
- Pharmacy Act
- Physiotherapy Act
- Prescription Monitoring Act
- Presumption of Death Act
- Professional Dietitians Act
- Psychologists Act
- Public Services Sustainability Act
- Queen Elizabeth II Health Sciences Centre Act
- Queen Elizabeth II Health Sciences Centre Expansion Act

- Registered Nurses Act
- Regulated Health Professions Network Act
- Respiratory Therapists Act
- Safer Needles in Healthcare Workplaces Act
- Support for Parents of Critically Ill or Abducted Children Act
- Tanning Beds Act
- Tobacco Access Act
- Tobacco Damages and Health-care Costs Recovery Act

References

Allin, S. (2008). Does equity in healthcare use vary across Canadian provinces? *Healthcare Policy, 3*(4), 83–99.

Angus Reid Institute. (2016). Premiers' performance. Available at http://angusreid.org/premier-approval-february2016/

Asada, Y., & Kephart, G. (2007). Equity in health services use and intensity of use in Canada. *BMC Health Services Research, 7*(41). https://doi.org/10.1186/1472-6963-7-41

Aubé, C. (2013). *Francophone and Acadian experiences in the primary health care system in Halifax, Nova Scotia* (Master's thesis). Dalhousie University, Halifax, Nova Scotia.

Aucoin, P. (1995). *The New Public Management: Canada in comparative perspective.* Montreal: Institute for Research on Public Policy.

Beck, M. (1957). *The government of Nova Scotia.* Toronto: University of Toronto Press. https://doi.org/10.3138/9781442656741

Berwick, D., Nolan, T., & Whittington, J. (2008). The triple aim: Care, health, and cost. *Health Affairs, 27*(3), 759–69. https://doi.org/10.1377/hlthaff.27.3.759

Bickerton, J. (1999). Reforming health care governance: The case of Nova Scotia. *Journal of Canadian Studies. Revue d'Etudes Canadiennes, 34*(2), 159–90. https://doi.org/10.3138/jcs.34.2.159

Black, M., & Fierlbeck, K. (2006). Whatever happened to regionalization? The curious case of Nova Scotia. *Canadian Public Administration, 49*(4), 506–26. https://doi.org/10.1111/j.1754-7121.2006.tb01996.x

Blake, D. (2001). Electoral democracy in the provinces. *IRPP Choices, 7*(2) March.

Bloom Program. (n.d.). The Bloom Program. Available at http://bloomprogram.ca

Boardman, A., Siemiatycki, M., & Vining, A. (2016). The theory and evidence concerning public-private partnerships in Canada and elsewhere. *University of Calgary School of Public Policy Research Papers 9*(12). Available at https://www.policyschool.ca/wp-content/uploads/2016/05/p3-boardman-siemiatycki-vining.pdf

Boase, J.P. (1994). *Shifting sands: Government-group relationships in the health care sector.* Montreal, Kingston: McGill-Queen's University Press.

Bowen, S. (2001). Language barriers in access to health care. Ottawa: Health Canada. Available at http://www.hc-sc.gc.ca/hcs-sss/pubs/acces/2001-lang-acces/index-eng.php

Bradley, S. (2016). Nova Scotia's drug monitoring program did not flag doctor charged with trafficking. *CBC News,* 25 February 2016. Available at http://www.cbc.ca/news/canada/nova-scotia/nova-scotia-drug-monitoring-doctor-1.3464409

Braveman, P.A., Egerter, S.A., Woolf, S.H., & Marks, J.S. (2011). When do we know enough to recommend action on the social determinants of health? *American Journal of Preventive Medicine, 40*(1), S58–66. https://doi.org/10.1016/j.amepre.2010.09.026

Bricker, D., & Ibbitson, J. (2013). *The big shift.* Toronto: Harper Collins.

Broten, L. (2014). Charting a path for growth: Nova Scotia tax and regulatory review. Available at http://www.novascotia.ca/finance/docs/tr/Tax_and_Regulatory_Review_Nov_2014.pdf

Buott, K. (2008). Decoding Corpus Sanchez. Nova Scotia Health Coalition. Available at http://nshealthcoalition.ca/column_decoding_corpus_sanchez/

Canada. (2013). Canadian tobacco, alcohol, and drugs survey. Available at https://www.canada.ca/en/health-canada/services/canadian-tobacco-alcohol-drugs-survey/2013-supplementary-tables.html

Canadian Midwifery Regulators Council. (2016). Midwifery in Canada. Available at http://cmrc-ccosf.ca/midwifery-canada

Canadian Agency for Drugs and Technologies in Health. (2015). The Canadian medical imaging inventory, 2015. Available at https://www.cadth.ca/canadian-medical-imaging-inventory-2015

Canadian Partnership against Cancer. (2016). Cancer system performance: Patient satisfaction. Available at http://www.systemperformance.ca/cancer-control-domain/person-centred-perspective/patient-satisfaction/

Canadian Society for Medical Laboratory Science. (2001). *Medical laboratory technologists national human resources review: A call to action.* Available at https://csmls.org/csmls/media/documents/publications/reports/csmls-hr-report.pdf

Cancer Care Nova Scotia. (2013). Navigating the cancer care system: Has the experience of African Nova Scotians improved? Available at http://

www.cancercare.ns.ca/site-cc/media/cancercare/ANS%20Report%20
April%202013%20Final.pdf

Capital District Health Authority. (2011). *The difference of primary health care: A report on the work of primary health care.* Halifax: Capital District Health Authority.

Capital District Health Authority. (2013). Annual report 2012–2013. Available at http://www.cdha.nshealth.ca/annual-report-2012-13/

Capital District Health Authority. (2014a). Patient Experience Reporting System annual report 2012–2013. Available at https://www.cdha.nshealth.ca/about-us/measuring-success-progress/patient-experience-survey

Capital District Health Authority. (2014b). Involving patients and citizens: A review of Capital Health's engagement policy achievements, 2010–2014.

Capital District Health Authority. (2014c). Blood collection services – Quality and patient safety. Available at http://www.cdha.nshealth.ca/pathology-laboratory-medicine/patient-information/blood-collection-services-quality-patient-safety

Capital District Health Authority. (2014d). Looking into the future: Capital Health 2013–14 annual report. Available at http://www.cdha.nshealth.ca/annual-report-2013-14/innovation.html

Carbert, L. (2015). Nova Scotia. In J. Wesley (Ed.), *Big worlds: Politics and elections in the Canadian provinces and territories* (pp. 36–58). Toronto: University of Toronto Press.

CBC. (2010). Telehealth line saved thousands of ER trips. Available at http://www.cbc.ca/news/canada/nova-scotia/telehealth-line-saved-thousands-of-er-trips-1.974791

CBC. (2014a). Janet Knox to lead newly merged health board. Available at http://www.cbc.ca/news/canada/nova-scotia/janet-knox-to-lead-newly-merged-health-board-1.2770382

CBC. (2014b). Liberals say no thanks to proposal from Nova Scotia health unions. Available at http://www.cbc.ca/news/canada/nova-scotia/liberals-say-no-thanks-to-proposal-from-nova-scotia-health-unions-1.2774487

CBC. (2015). James Dorsey fired for a fourth time as health arbitrator. Available at http://www.cbc.ca/news/canada/nova-scotia/james-dorsey-fired-for-a-fourth-time-as-health-arbitrator-1.2974520

Chiu, E. (2016). Dr. Sarah Jones review calls for ban on doctors picking up prescriptions. *CBC News*, 27 October 2016. Available at http://www.cbc.ca/news/canada/nova-scotia/sarah-jones-review-prescription-drug-monitoring-1.3824203

CIHI. (n.d.). Your Health System (interactive website). Available at http://yourhealthsystem.cihi.ca

CIHI. (2011). *Health care cost drivers: The facts.* Ottawa: Canadian Institute for Health Information. Available at https://secure.cihi.ca/free_products /health_care_cost_drivers_the_facts_en.pdf.

CIHI. (2012a). *All-cause readmission to acute care and return to the emergency department.* Ottawa: Canadian Institute for Health Information. Available at https://secure.cihi.ca/free_products/Readmission_to_acutecare_en.pdf

CIHI. (2012b). *Highlights of 2010–2011 inpatient hospitalizations and emergency department visits.* Ottawa: Canadian Institute for Health Information. Available at https://secure.cihi.ca/free_products/DAD-NACRS_Highlights _2010-2011_EN.pdf

CIHI. (2013). *Prescribed drug spending in Canada, 2013: A focus on public drug programs.* Ottawa: Canadian Institute for Health Information.

CIHI. (2014). *National health expenditure trends 1975–2014.* Ottawa: Canadian Institute for Health Information.

CIHI. (2015a). *National health expenditure trends 1975–2015.* Ottawa: Canadian Institute for Health Information.

CIHI. (2015b). Physician services benefit rates report, Canada, 2013–2014. Ottawa: Canadian Institute for Health Information. Available at https:// secure.cihi.ca/free_products/PSBR-2013_2014_EN_web.pdf

CIHI. (2015c). *Public sector health expenditure by use of funds (by province).* Available at https://www.cihi.ca/en/spending-and-health-workforce/spending /national-health-expenditure-trends

CIHI. (2016a). *National health expenditure trends 1975–2015.* Ottawa: Canadian Institute for Health Information.

CIHI. (2016b). National Physician Database 2014–15. Available at https:// secure.cihi.ca/estore/productSeries.htm?pc=PCC476

CIHI. (2016c). Wait times for priority procedures in Canada, 2016. Available at https://secure.cihi.ca/estore/productFamily.htm?locale=en&pf=PFC3108

CIHI. (2016d). Supply, distribution, and migration of Canadian physicians, (data tables). Available at https://secure.cihi.ca/estore/productSeries.htm?pc=PCC34

CIHI. (2017). National health expenditure trends. Data tables on health spending. Available at https://www.cihi.ca/en/national-health-expenditure-trends

CMA. (2015). Canadian Physician Statistics. Available at https://www.cma.ca /En/Pages/canadian-physician-statistics.aspx

Colbert, Y. (2015). Nova Scotia walk-in clinics face doctor limits. *CBC News,* 2 December 2015. Available at http://www.cbc.ca/news/canada/nova-scotia /nova-scotia-walk-in-clinics-1.3345938

Colbert, Y. (2016). Nova Scotia spends $39M on electronic medical records push. *CBC News,* 13 April 2016. Available at http://www.cbc.ca/news /canada/nova-scotia/medical-care-records-expense-1.3530728

College of Dental Hygienists of Nova Scotia. (2014). *Dental hygienists prevent more to treat less* (White Paper). Available at http://www.nsrhpn.ca/wp-content /uploads/2014/08/Prevent-More-to-Treat-Less-OCTOBER-2-FINAL.pdf

College of Physicians and Surgeons of Nova Scotia. (2013). Guidelines regarding conflict of interest. Available at http://www.cpsns.ns.ca /DesktopModules/Bring2mind/DMX/Download.aspx?PortalId=0&TabId=1 29&EntryId=37

College of Physicians and Surgeons of Nova Scotia. (2014). Professional standard and guidelines on complementary and alternative therapies. Available at http://www.cpsns.ns.ca/DesktopModules/Bring2mind/DMX /Download.aspx?PortalId=0&TabId=129&EntryId=48

Community Foundations of Nova Scotia. (2011). *Nova Scotia's vital signs.* Available at https://issuu.com/communityfoundationsofcanada/docs/novascotia_2011

Corfu, N. (2017). Halifax doctor ties health-care woes to poor use of medical professionals. CBC News, 8 November 2017. Available at http://www.cbc.ca /news/canada/nova-scotia/john-ross-healthcare-doctor-shortage-waitlist -creativity-paramedics-nurses-1.4393000

Côté-Sergent, A., Échevin, D., & Michaud, P.C. (2016). The concentration of hospital-based medical spending: Evidence from Canada. *Fiscal Studies, 37*(3–4), 627–51. https://doi.org/10.1111/j.1475-5890.2016.12125

Coyte, P.C., & McKeever, P. (2001). Home care in Canada: Passing the buck. *Canadian Journal of Nursing Research, 33*(2), 11–25.

Deber, R. (2008). Access without appropriateness: Chicken Little in charge? *Healthcare Policy, 4*(1), 23–9.

Denis, J.L., Brown, L., Forest, P.G., Normandin, J.M., Cambourieu, C., Cannizzaro, V., & Preval, J. (2015). Policy capacity for health system reform. Report submitted to Nova Scotia Health Research Foundation. http:// archives.enap.ca/bibliotheques/2015/11/031003060.pdf

Denis, J.L., Contandriopoulos, D., & Beaulieu, M.D. (2004). Regionalization in Canada: A promising heritage to build on. *Healthcare Papers, 5*(1), 12–31.

Doctors Nova Scotia. (2015). Electronic medical records. Available at http:// www.doctorsns.com/en/home/practiceresources/electronic-medical -records/default.aspx

Dolan, D., Grainger, N., MacCallum, N., Creatura, D., Forrester, J., & Shiller, S. (2012). The Institute for Clinical Evaluative Sciences: 20 years and counting. *Healthcare Quarterly, 15*(4), 19–21. https://doi.org/10.12927/hcq.2012.23194

Dorsey, J. (2015). Mediation-arbitration decision under the Health Authorities Act 2014. Halifax, Nova Scotia, 17 January 2015.

Duckett, S. (2015). Alberta: Health spending in the land of plenty. In G. Marchildon and L. di Matteo (Eds.), *Bending the cost curve in health care:*

Canada's provinces in international perspective (pp. 297–326). Toronto: University of Toronto Press.

Duckett, S. (2016). Regionalization as one manifestation of the pursuit of the Holy Grail. *Healthcare Papers, 16*(1), 53–7. https://doi.org/10.12927/hcpap.2016.24770

Employment and Development Canada. (2012). Labour market bulletin: Nova Scotia, October 2012 (annual report).

Employment and Development Canada. (2013). Labour market bulletin: Nova Scotia, October 2013 (quarterly report).

Epstein, H. *Rise again: Nova Scotia's NDP On the rocks*. Halifax: Empty Mirrors Press, 2015.

Evans, G.W., & Cassells, R.C. (2013). Childhood poverty, cumulative risk exposure, and mental health in emerging adults. *Clinical Psychological Science, 2*(3), 287–96. https://doi.org/10.1177/2167702613501496

Evans, R.G. (2011). The sorcerer's apprentices. *Healthcare Policy, 7*(2), 14–22.

Evans, R.G., & McGrail, K.M. (2008). Richard III, Barer-Stoddart and the daughter of time. *Healthcare Policy, 3*(3), 18–28.

Evans, R.G., McGrail, K.M., Morgan, S.G., Barer, M.L., & Hertzman, C. (2001). Apocalypse no: Population aging and the future of health care systems. *Canadian Journal on Aging, 20*(S1), 160–91. https://doi.org/10.1017/S0714980800015282

Fafard, P. (2015). Beyond the usual suspects: Using political science to enhance public health policy making. *Journal of Epidemiology and Community Health, 69*(11), 1129–32. https://doi.org/10.1136/jech-2014-204608

Fiandt, K. (2006). The chronic care model: Description and application for practice. *Topics in Advanced Practice Nursing eJournal 6*(4).

Fierlbeck, K. (2011). *Health care in Canada*. Toronto: University of Toronto Press.

Fierlbeck, K. (2016). The politics of regionalization. *Healthcare Papers, 16*(1), 58–62. https://doi.org/10.12927/hcpap.2016.24772

Finance Canada. (2016). Federal support to provinces and territories. Available at http://www.fin.gc.ca/fedprov/mtp-eng.asp

Fingard, J., & Rutherford, J. (2005). The politics of mental health care in Nova Scotia: The case of the Halifax County Hospital, 1940–1976. *Acadiensis, 35*(1). Available at https://journals.lib.unb.ca/index.php/acadiensis/article/view/10617/11243

Fingard, J., & Rutherford, J. (2011). Deinstitutionalization and vocational rehabilitation for mental health consumers in Nova Scotia since the 1950s. *Social History, 44*(88), 385–408. https://doi.org/10.1353/his.2011.0019

Fortune. (2009). Fortune 500, 2009. Available at http://fortune.com/fortune500/2009/exxon-mobil-corporation-1/

Fraser, F.M. (1961). The Maritime Medical Care Plan. *Canadian Journal of Public Health*, *52*(5), 206–13.

Fries, J. (1980). Aging, natural death, and the compression of morbidity. *New England Journal of Medicine*, *303*(3), 130–5. https://doi.org/10.1056/NEJM198007173030304

Furlan, A.D., MacDougall, P., Pellerin, D., Shaw, K., Spitzig, D., Wilson, G., & Wright, J. (2014). Overview of four prescription monitoring review programs in Canada. *Pain Research & Management*, *19*(2), 102–6. https://doi.org/10.1155/2014/634171

Galloway, G. (2016). Canadians differ from Trump on view of public health care, poll shows. *Globe and Mail*, 14 November 2016. Available at https://www.theglobeandmail.com/news/politics/canadians-differ-from-trump-on-health-care-poll-shows/article32835912/

Gorman, M. (2014). "A longer path" to savings from health board mergers, Glavine admits. *Chronicle Herald*, 26 June 2014. Available at http://thechronicleherald.ca/novascotia/1218499-a-longer-path-to-savings-from-health-board-mergers-glavine-admits

Gorman, M. (2015). $3.37m in unreleased health merger costs angers opposition. *Chronicle Herald*, 16 November 2015. Available at http://thechronicleherald.ca/novascotia/1322659-3.37m-in-unreleased-health-merger-costs-angers-opposition

Gorman, M. (2016a). Nurse practitioners could replace doctors at some walk-in clinics. *CBC News*, 16 June 2016. Available at http://www.cbc.ca/news/canada/nova-scotia/health-care-nova-scotia-nurse-practitioners-walk-in-clinics-1.3636697

Gorman, M. (2016b). Who's watching out for the patients? *Halifax Examiner*, 18 February 2016. Available at https://www.halifaxexaminer.ca/province-house/whos-watching-out-for-patients/

Grant, K.R., Amaratunga, C., Armstrong, P., Boscoe, M., Pederson, A., & Willson, K. (Eds.). (2004). *Caring for/caring about: Women, home care, and unpaid caregiving*. Toronto: University of Toronto Press.

Greer, S.L. (forthcoming). Health policy and territorial politics: Disciplinary misunderstandings and directions for research. In E. Hepburn and K. Detterbeck (Eds.), *Edward Elgar handbook of territorial politics*. Cheltenham, U.K.: Edward Elgar Press. Available at https://deepblue.lib.umich.edu/bitstream/handle/2027.42/136224/Health%20and%20territorial%20politics.pdf?sequence=1&isAllowed=y

Hajizadeh, M. (2017). Does socioeconomic status affect length wait time in Canada: Evidence from Canadian community health surveys. *European Journal of Health Economics*. https://doi.org/10.1007/s10198-017-0889-3

Hassenteufel, P., Smyrl M., Genieys W., & Moreno-Fuentes FJ. (2010). Programmatic actors and the transformation of European health care states. *Journal of Health Politics, Policy and Law, 35*, 517–38.

Health Association of Nova Scotia. (2014). Rising to the challenge: Responding to increasing demands in home care. Available at http://caregiversns.org/images /uploads/Responding_to_the_Challenge_Report_-_FINAL_July_7_2014.pdf

Henry, D.A., Schultz, S.E., Glazier, R.H., Bhatia, R.S., Dhalla, I.A., & Laupacis, A. (2012). *Payments to Ontario physicians from Ministry of Health and long term care sources, 1992/93 to 2009/10. ICES Investigative Report.* Toronto: Institute for Clinical Evaluative Sciences.

Hirdes, J. (2001). Long-term funding in Canada: A policy mosaic. *Journal of Aging & Social Policy, 13*(2–3), 69–81.

Howe, M. (2013). Nova Scotia's handling of electronic medical reports industry leaves competitors feeling ill. *Halifax Media Co-op*, 18 April 2013. Available at http://halifax.mediacoop.ca/fr/story/nova-scotias-handling-electronic -medical-reports-i/17185.

Hospice Society of Greater Halifax. (2013). Hospice care gap in Nova Scotia. Available at http://www.ehospice.com/canadaenglish/Default /tabid/10678/ArticleId/5015

Human Resources Development Canada. (2003). *A study of health human resources in Nova Scotia 2003.* Halifax: Health Care Human Resource Sector Council. Available at http://tools.hhr-rhs.ca/index.php?option=com _mtree&task=att_download&link_id=5201&cf_id=68&lang=en

Hurley, J., Lomas J., & Bhatia, V. (1994). When tinkering is not enough: Provincial reform to manage health care resources. *Canadian Public Administration, 37*(3), 490–514.

Hutchison, B. (2008). A long time coming: Primary healthcare renewal in Canada. *Healthcare Papers, 8*(2), 10–24. https://doi.org/10.12927 /hcpap.2008.19704

Hutchison, B., Abelson, J., & Lavis, J. (2001). Primary care in Canada: So much innovation, so little change. *Health Affairs, 20*(3), 116–31. https:// doi.org/10.1377/hlthaff.20.3.116

Jensen, J., Travers, A.H., Marshall, E.G., Leadlay, S., & Carter, A.J.E. (2014). Insights into the implementation and operation of a novel paramedic long-term care program. *Prehospital Emergency Care, 18*(1), 86–91. https:// doi.org/10.3109/10903127.2013.831506

Jin, M., Naumann, T., Regier, L., Bugden, S., Allen, M., Salach, L., . . ., & Dolovich, L. (2012). A brief review of academic detailing in Canada: Another role for pharmacists. *Canadian Pharmacists Journal, 145*(3), 142–6.e2. https:// doi.org/10.3821/145.3.cpj142

Kephart, G., Asada, Y., Atherton, F., Burge, F., Campbell, L.A., Campbell, M., . . ., & Terashima, M. (2016). *Small area variation in rates of high-cost healthcare use across Nova Scotia.* Halifax: Maritime SPOR SUPPORT Unit.

Kephart, G., Thomas, V.S., & Maclean, D.R. (1998). Socioeconomic differences in the use of physician services in Nova Scotia. *American Journal of Public Health, 88*(5), 800–3. https://doi.org/10.2105/AJPH.88.5.800

Kisely, S., Terashima, M., & Langille, D. (2008). A population-based analysis of the health experience of African Nova Scotians. *Canadian Medical Association Journal, 179*(7), 653–8. https://doi.org/10.1503/cmaj.071279

Klein, D., Brown, A., Huynh, T., Bevan, G., Markel, F., Ottaway, S., . . ., & Zyblock, M. (2013). *Capital spending in healthcare: A missed opportunity for improvement?* Canadian Foundation for Healthcare Improvement. Available at http://www.cfhi-fcass.ca/Libraries/Reports/Capital-Spending-Brown-E.sflb.ashx.

Koon, A., Hawkins, B., & Mayhew, S. (2016). Framing and the health policy process: A scoping review. *Health Policy and Planning, 31*(6), 801–16. https://doi.org/10.1093/heapol/czv128

Lahey, W. (2013). Legislating interprofessional regulatory collaboration in Nova Scotia. *Health Reform Observer, 1*(1). https://doi.org/10.13162/hro-ors.01.01.04

Lahey, W., & Fierlbeck, K. (2016). Legislating collaborative self-regulation in Canada: A comparative policy analysis. *Journal of Interprofessional Care, 30*(2), 211–16. https://doi.org/10.3109/13561820.2015.1109501

Laroche, J. (2017). Internal report recommends closing inpatient detox units, converting others. *CBC News,* 7 March 2017. Available at http://www.cbc.ca/news/canada/nova-scotia/mental-health-addictions-detox-beds-day-clinics-report-1.4011901

Law, M., Heard, D., Fisher, J., Douillard, J., Muzika, G., & Sketris, I. (2013). The geographic accessibility of pharmacies in Nova Scotia. *Canadian Pharmacists Journal, 146*(1), 39–46. https://doi.org/10.1177/1715163512473062

Lazar, H., Lavis, J., Forest, P.G., & Church, J. (2013). *Paradigm freeze: Why is it so hard to reform health-care policy in Canada.* Montreal, Kingston: Institute of Intergovernmental Relations and McGill-Queen's University Press.

Leonard, P., & Sweetman, A. (2015). Paying the health workforce. In G. Marchildon & L. di Matteo (Eds.), *Bending the cost curve in health care: Canada's provinces in international perspective* (pp. 139–67). Toronto: University of Toronto Press.

Levert, S. (2013). *Sustainability of the Canadian health care system and impact of the 2014 revision to the Canada Health Transfer.* Canadian Institute of Actuaries and Society of Actuaries. Available at http://www.cia-ica.ca/docs/default-source/2013/213075e.pdf

Levy A., McDonald, T., Krause, J., Anderson, D. (2015). Patient-oriented research a key to better service. *Chronicle-Herald*, 13 June 2015: F4.

Leighton, A.L. (1982). *Caring for mentally ill people: Psychological and social barriers in historical context.* Cambridge: Cambridge University Press.

Lewis, S., & Kouri, D. (2004). Regionalization: Making sense of the Canadian experience. *Healthcare Papers*, 5(1), 12–31. https://doi.org/10.12927/hcpap.2004.16847

Liberal Party of Nova Scotia. (2013). Nova Scotia First: Nova Scotia Liberal Party Platform 2013. Available at http://www.liberal.ns.ca/wp-content/uploads/2013/09/2013-Liberal-Platform.pdf

Lomas, J. (1996). Devolved authorities in Canada: The new site of health-care system conflict? In J.L. Dorland & S.M. Davis (Eds.), *How many roads? Regionalization and decentralization in health care* (pp. 26–34). Kingston: Queen's University School of Policy Studies.

Lomas, J. (2003). Past concerns and future roles for regional health boards. *Canadian Medical Association Journal*, 164(3), 356–7.

MacLennan, N. (2016). First Nations communities health data hints at high rates of diabetes. *CBC News*, 30 March 2016. Available at http://www.cbc.ca/news/canada/nova-scotia/first-nations-health-data-diabetes-heart-attacks-1.3511103

MacLeod, J. (2006). Nova Scotia politics: Clientelism and John Savage. *Canadian Journal of Political Science*, 39(3), 553–70. https://doi.org/10.1017/S0008423906060276

Marble, A.E. (1993). *Surgeons, smallpox, and the poor: A history of medicine and social conditions in Nova Scotia, 1749–1799.* Montreal, Kingston: McGill-Queens University Press.

Marble, A.E. (2006). *Physicians, pestilence, and the poor: A history and social conditions in Nova Scotia, 1800–1867.* Victoria, BC: Trafford Publishing.

Marchildon, G.P. (2013). *Health systems in transition: Canada* (2nd ed.). Toronto: University of Toronto Press.

Marchildon, G.P. (2015). The crisis of regionalization. *Healthcare Management Forum*, 28(6), 236–8. https://doi.org/10.1177/0840470415599115

Marchildon, G.P. (2016). Regionalization: What have we learned? *Healthcare Papers*, 16(1), 8–14. https://doi.org/10.12927/hcpap.2016.24766

Marmor, T., & Wendt, C. (2012). Conceptual frameworks for comparing healthcare politics and policy. *Health Policy (Amsterdam)*, 107(1), 11–20. https://doi.org/10.1016/j.healthpol.2012.06.003

Mathieson, C.M., Bailey, N., & Gurevich, M. (2002). Health care services for lesbian and bisexual women: Some Canadian data. *Health Care for Women International*, 23(2), 185–96.

McAlister, C., & Twohig, P. (2005). The check-off: A precursor of medicare in Canada. *Canadian Medical Association Journal, 173*(12), 1504–6.

McKee, M., Edwards, N., & Atun, R. (2006). Public-private partnerships for hospitals. *Bulletin of the World Health Organization, 84*(11), 890–4.

Mi'kmaq Health Research Group. (2007). *The health of the Nova Scotia Mi'kmaq population.* Union of Nova Scotia Indians. Available at http://www.unsi.ns.ca/wp-content/uploads/2015/07/ns-rhs-report-07.pdf

Morgan, S., Law, M., Daw, J., Abraham, L., & Martin, D. (2015). Estimated cost of universal public coverage of prescription drugs in Canada. *Canadian Medical Association Journal, 187*(7), 491–7. https://doi.org/10.1503/cmaj.141564

Mossialos, E., Courtin, E., Naci, H., Benrimoj, S., Bouvy, M., Farris, K., . . ., & Sketris, I. (2015). From "retailers" to health care providers: Transforming the role of community pharmacists in chronic disease management. *Health Policy (Amsterdam), 119*(5), 628–39. https://doi.org/10.1016/j.healthpol.2015.02.007

Muldoon, L.K., Hogg, W.E., & Levitt, M. (2006). Primary care (PC) and primary health care (PHC): What is the difference? *Canadian Journal of Public Health, 97*(5), 409–11.

Nova Scotia. (1950). *Report on the survey of hospitals in Nova Scotia under the Federal Health Survey Grant.* Halifax, Nova Scotia.

Nova Scotia. (1967). *Report of the Medical Care Insurance Advisory Commission.* Halifax, Nova Scotia.

Nova Scotia. (1972). *Health care in Nova Scotia: A new direction for the seventies* (Report of the Nova Scotia Council of Health). Halifax, Nova Scotia.

Nova Scotia. (1989). *Report of the Nova Scotia Royal Commission on Health Care* (Gallant report). Halifax, Nova Scotia.

Nova Scotia. (1994). *Nova Scotia's blueprint for health system reform:Minister's Action Committee on Health Care Reform* (Blueprint Committee Report). Halifax, Nova Scotia.

Nova Scotia. (1999). *Minister's Task Force on Regionalized Health Care in Nova Scotia: Final report and recommendations* (Goldbloom report). Halifax, Nova Scotia.

Nova Scotia. (2006). *Continuing care strategy for Nova Scotia: Shaping the future of continuing care.* Available at http://www.healthteamnovascotia.ca/files/Continuing_Care_Strategy06.pdf

Nova Scotia. (2007a). *Changing Nova Scotia's healthcare system: Creating sustainability through transformation.* Commissioned from Corpus Sanchez Consultants. Available at https://novascotia.ca/dhw/publications/Provincial_Health_Services_Operational_Review_Report.pdf

Nova Scotia. (2007b). *Nova Scotia's Nursing Strategy: Ensuring a healthy, vibrant nursing community.* Available at http://www.healthteamnovascotia.ca/files /Nurses%20Advisory%20Brochure_lowres.pdf

Nova Scotia. (2010a, October). *The patient journey through emergency care in Nova Scotia: A prescription for new medicine.* Prepared by John Ross. Available at http://novascotia.ca/dhw/publications/Dr-Ross-The-Patient-Journey -Through-Emergency-Care-in-Nova-Scotia.pdf

Nova Scotia. (2010b, December). *Better care sooner: The plan to improve emergency care.* Available at http://novascotia.ca/dhw/publications/Dr-Ross-The -Patient-Journey-Through-Emergency-Care-in-Nova-Scotia.pdf

Nova Scotia. (2010c). *Model of Care Initiative in Nova Scotia (MOCINS): Final evaluation report.* Commissioned from the WHO Collaborating Centre on Health Workforce Planning and Research. Available at http://novascotia.ca /dhw/mocins/docs/MOCINS-evaluation-report.pdf

Nova Scotia. (2010d). *Aboriginal long term care in Nova Scotia.* Available at http:// novascotia.ca/dhw/ccs/documents/Aboriginal-Long-Term-Care-in-Nova -Scotia.pdf

Nova Scotia. (2011). *A summary of the current state of mental health and addictions services in Nova Scotia.* Available at http://www.nshrf.ca/sites/default/files /mental_health_and_addictions_summary_document_09.14.11.pdf

Nova Scotia. (2012a). *Shaping our physician workforce.* Available at http:// novascotia.ca/dhw/publications/Physician_Resource_Plan_Shaping_our _physician_Workforce.pdf

Nova Scotia. (2012b). *Come together: Report and recommendations of the Mental Health and Addictions Strategy Advisory Committee.* Available at http:// 0-nsleg-edeposit.gov.ns.ca.legcat.gov.ns.ca/deposit/b10647934.pdf

Nova Scotia. (2012c). *2012–2013 Continuing care resource guide for First Nations communities in Nova Scotia* (a report of the Nova Scotia Aboriginal Continuing Care Policy Forum). Halifax, Nova Scotia.

Nova Scotia. (2014a). *Now or never: An urgent call to action for Nova Scotians* (the Report of the Nova Scotia Commission on Building our New Economy). Halifax, Nova Scotia. Available at https://onens.ca/img/now-or-never.pdf

Nova Scotia. (2014b). *Care right now: Evaluating the collaborative emergency centre experience in Nova Scotia.* Report prepared by Stylus Consulting. Available at http://novascotia.ca/DHW/publications/Care-Right-Now-Evaluating-the -CEC-Experience-in-Nova-Scotia-Full-Report.pdf

Nova Scotia. (2014c). *Physician recruitment and retention action team report.* Available at http://novascotia.ca/dhw/publications/Physician-Recruitment -Retention-Action-Team-Report.pdf

Nova Scotia. (2014d). *Integrated palliative care: Planning for action in Nova Scotia.* Available at https://novascotia.ca/dhw/palliativecare/documents /Integrated-Palliative-Care-Strategy.pdf

Nova Scotia. (2014e). Thrive! A Plan for a Healthier Nova Scotia. Available at https://thrive.novascotia.ca/

Nova Scotia. (2014f). *Health care conversations: What we heard.* Available at http://0-nsleg-edeposit.gov.ns.ca.legcat.gov.ns.ca/deposit/b10672084.pdf

Nova Scotia. (2015a). Nova Scotia Wait Times (website). http:// waittimes.novascotia.ca/

Nova Scotia. (2015b). Continuing care, 2006 strategy evaluation. Executive summary June 2015. Halifax, Nova Scotia.

Nova Scotia. (2015c). Province of Nova Scotia public accounts, volume 1: Consolidated financial statements. Available at http://www.novascotia.ca /finance/site-finance/media/finance/PublicAccounts2015/2015_Vol1.pdf

Nova Scotia. (2016a). Budget 2016–2017: Estimates and supplementary detail. Available at http://www.novascotia.ca/finance/site-finance/media/finance /budget2016/Estimates-and-Supplementary-Detail.pdf

Nova Scotia. (2016b). Province of Nova Scotia public accounts, volume 1: Consolidated financial statements. Available at https://www.novascotia.ca /finance/site-finance/media/finance/PublicAccounts2016/2016_Vol1.pdf

Nova Scotia Archives. (2016a). African Nova Scotians in the age of slavery and abolition. Available at https://novascotia.ca/archives/africanns/results.asp ?Search=&SearchList1=1&Language=English

Nova Scotia Archives. (2016b). Gone but never forgotten: Bob Brooks' photographic portrait of Africville in the 1960s. Available at https:// novascotia.ca/archives/africville/

Nova Scotia Department of Finance. (2000). Public Accounts for 2000. http:// www.novascotia.ca/finance/en/home/publications/publicaccounts/default.aspx

Nova Scotia Department of Finance. (2010). Public Accounts for 2010. http:// www.novascotia.ca/ finance/en/home/publications/publicaccounts/default.aspx

Nova Scotia Department of Finance. (2013). Nova Scotia economic indicators, 12 August 2013. Available at http://www.novascotia.ca/finance/publish/EI /NSEI1308.PDF

Nova Scotia Department of Finance. (2014a). Employment Insurance (EI), Nova Scotia. Available at http://www.novascotia.ca/finance/statistics /media/EIJuly_NovaScotia.png

Nova Scotia Department of Finance. (2014b). Public Accounts for 2014. http://www.novascotia.ca/finance/en/home/publications/publicaccounts /default.aspx

Nova Scotia Department of Health. (2005). Province signs 10-year contract with Medavie Blue Cross. Available at http://novascotia.ca/news/release/?id=20050729006

Nova Scotia Department of Health. (2006a). *A primary health care evaluation system for Nova Scotia.* Commissioned from Pyra Management Consulting Services, Research Power Incorporated. Available at https://novascotia.ca/dhw/publications/Primary-Health-Care-Evaluation-Report-2006.pdf

Nova Scotia Department of Health. (2006b). *The renewal of public health in Nova Scotia: Building a public health system to meet the needs of Nova Scotians.* Available at https://novascotia.ca/dhw/publichealth/documents/Renewal-of-Public-Health-Report.pdf

Nova Scotia Department of Health. (2007). *Nova Scotia's nursing strategy: Summary report 2001–2006.* Available at http://www.healthteamnovascotia.ca/files/Nursing_Strategy_Summary_2001_2006.pdf

Nova Scotia Department of Health. (2010). *Nova Scotia's response to H1N1: A summary report.* Available at http://novascotia.ca/dhw/publications/H1N1-Summary-Report.pdf

Nova Scotia Department of Health and Wellness. (2009). *Model of Care Initiative in Nova Scotia: Phase I implementation status report.* Prepared by K. Fraser and C. Cruikshank. Available at http://novascotia.ca/dhw/mocins/docs/MOCINS%20Phase%20I%20Implementation%20Report.pdf

Nova Scotia Department of Health and Wellness. (2010). *Better care sooner: The plan to improve emergency care.* Available at http://novascotia.ca/dhw/publications/Better-Care-Sooner-plan.pdf

Nova Scotia Department of Health and Wellness. (2011). *Midwifery in Nova Scotia: Report of the external assessment.* Prepared by K. Kaufman, K. Robinson, K. Buhler, and G. Hazlit. Available at http://0-nsleg-edeposit.gov.ns.ca.legcat.gov.ns.ca/deposit/b10633121.pdf

Nova Scotia Department of Health and Wellness. (2012a). *Physician resource planning: A recommended model and implementation framework.* Commissioned by Social Sector Metrics Inc. and Health Intelligence Inc. Available at http://www.doctorsns.com/site/media/DoctorsNS/PhysicianResourcePlanning-finalreport.pdf

Nova Scotia Department of Health and Wellness. (2012b). *The renewal of public health in Nova Scotia: Mid-course review.* Available at http://novascotia.ca/dhw/publications/Mid_Course_Review_Feb2012.pdf

Nova Scotia Department of Health and Wellness. (2014). *Accountability report 2013–2014.* Available at http://novascotia.ca/dhw/corporate-reports/documents/Accountibility-Report-2013-2014-DHW.pdf

Nova Scotia Department of Health and Wellness. (2015a). *Nova Scotia health profile 2015.* Available at http://novascotia.ca/dhw/publichealth/documents/Population-Health-Profile-Nova-Scotia.pdf

Nova Scotia Department of Health and Wellness. (2015b). *Oral Health Advisory Group, Phase 1: Report to the Minister of Health and Wellness*. Available at http://novascotia.ca/dhw/publications/Oral-Health-Advisory-Group-Phase-1-Report-to-the-Minister.pdf

Nova Scotia Department of Health and Wellness. (2015c). Government will introduce legislation to determine health-care representation (press release). 20 February 2015. Available at http://novascotia.ca/news/release/?id=20150220002

Nova Scotia Department of Health and Wellness. (2015d). Statement of mandate 2015–2016. Available at https://beta.novascotia.ca/sites/default/files/documents/2015-2016-DHW-Statement-of-Mandate.pdf

Nova Scotia Department of Health and Wellness. (2015e). *Accountability report 2014–2015*. Available at https://novascotia.ca/government/accountability/

Nova Scotia Department of Health and Wellness. (2016a). *Outcomes evaluation of the Bloom Program*. Prepared by L. Jacobs, D. Gardner, A. Murphy.

Nova Scotia Department of Health and Wellness. (2016b). Lower Seniors' Pharmacare premiums begin April 1st (press release). 15 January 2016. Available at http://novascotia.ca/news/release/?id=20160115003

Nova Scotia Department of Health and Wellness. (2016c). *Accountability report 2015–2016*. Available at https://novascotia.ca/government/accountability/2015-2016/2015-2016-Health-and-Wellness-Accountability.pdf

Nova Scotia Hansard. (2002). Committee on Public Accounts, 30 January 2002. Available at http://nslegislature.ca/index.php/committees/committee_hansard/C7/pa020130

Nova Scotia Hansard. (2013). House of Assembly, Debates of May 1st, 2013. Available at http://www.openhousens.ca/debates/debates-1-may-2013/?page=9

Nova Scotia Hansard. (2014). Committee on Human Resources. 16 December 2014. Available at http://nslegislature.ca/index.php/committees/committee_hansard/C8/hr2014dec16

Nova Scotia Hansard. (2015a). Committee on Public Accounts. 18 February 2015. Available at http://nslegislature.ca/index.php/committees/committee_hansard/C7/pa2015feb18

Nova Scotia Hansard. (2015b). Committee on Public Accounts. 13 May 2015. Available at http://nslegislature.ca/index.php/committees/committee_hansard/C7/pa2015may13

Nova Scotia Health Authority. (2015a). *NSHA Business Plan 2015–16*. Available at http://www.nshealth.ca/sites/nshealth.ca/files/2015-16_nsha_business_plan_-_master_final_2015-06-03.pdf

Nova Scotia Health Authority. (2015b). Administrative manual, policy and procedures. Available at http://policy.nshealth.ca/Site_Published/nsha/document_render.aspx?documentRender.IdType=6&documentRender.GenericField=&documentRender.Id=54156

Nova Scotia Health Research Foundation. (2009). *Major health issues in Nova Scotia: An environmental scan.* Available at http://www.nshrf.ca/sites/default/files/environmental_scan_-current_major_health_issues.pdf

Nova Scotia Hospice Palliative Care Association. (n.d.). (website) nshpca.ca/wp-content/uploads/resources/advocacy/campaignads.pdf

Nova Scotia Medical Services Insurance. (2014). *Physicians' manual.* Available at http://www.medavie.bluecross.ca/static/MSI/PhysicianManual.pdf

Nova Scotia Medical Society. (1960). Editorial: The price of freedom. *The Nova Scotia Medical Bulletin, 39*(8), 1.

Nova Scotia Office of the Auditor General. (1999). *Report of Auditor General 1999,* chapter 7, Northern Regional Health Board and follow-up to 1998 comments on RHBs and NDOs. Available at http://oag-ns.ca/publications/1999

Nova Scotia Office of the Auditor General. (2000). *Report of the Auditor General 2000,* chapter 8, Emergency health services. Available at http://oag-ns.ca/publications/2000

Nova Scotia Office of the Auditor General. (2004). *Report of the Auditor General December 2004,* chapter 7, Pharmacare and other drug programs. Available at http://oag-ns.ca/publications/2004

Nova Scotia Office of the Auditor General. (2005). *Report of the Auditor General, June 2005,* chapter 6, Nova Scotia hospital information system program. Available at http://oag-ns.ca/publications/2005

Nova Scotia Office of the Auditor General. (2007). *Report of the Auditor General, June 2007,* chapter 3, Emergency health services. Available at http://oag-ns.ca/publications/2007

Nova Scotia Office of the Auditor General. (2010a). *Report of the Auditor General, June 2010,* chapter 4, Mental health services. Available at http://oag-ns.ca/publications/2010

Nova Scotia Office of the Auditor General. (2010b). *Report of the Auditor General, February 2010,* chapter 3, Education: Contract management of public-private schools. Available at http://oag-ns.ca/publications/2010

Nova Scotia Office of the Auditor General. (2011). *Report of the Auditor General, May 2011,* chapter 5, Long term care – New and replacement facilities. Available at http://oag-ns.ca/publications/2011

Nova Scotia Office of the Auditor General. (2012a). *Report of the Auditor General, May 2012,* chapter 3, Addiction services at Annapolis Valley Health. Available at https://www.oag-ns.ca/publications/2012

Nova Scotia Office of the Auditor General. (2012b). *Report of the Auditor General, May 2012,* chapter 5, Nova Scotia Prescription Monitoring Program. Available at http://oag-ns.ca/publications/2012

Nova Scotia Office of the Auditor General, (2012c). *Report of the Auditor General, November 2012*, chapter 4, Hospital system capital planning. Available at http://oag-ns.ca/publications/2012

Nova Scotia Office of the Auditor General. (2013). *Report of the Auditor General, November 2013*, chapter 4, Public health surveillance. Available at http://oag-ns.ca/publications/2013

Nova Scotia Office of the Auditor General. (2014a). *Report of the Auditor General, January 2014*, chapter 4, Indicators of financial condition. Available at http://oag-ns.ca/publications/2014 pdf

Nova Scotia Office of the Auditor General. (2014b). *Report of the Auditor General, May 2014*, chapter 6, Physician alternative funding arrangements. Available at http://oag-ns.ca/publications/2014

Nova Scotia Office of the Auditor General. (2014c). *Report of the Auditor General, December 2014*, chapter 4, Surgical waitlist and operating room utilization. Available at https://www.oag-ns.ca/publications/2014

Nova Scotia Office of the Auditor General. (2016a). *Report of the Auditor General, June 2016*, chapter 1, Homes for special care: Identification and management of health and safety risks. Available at http://oag-ns.ca/sites/default/files/publications/Chapter%201_0.pdf

Nova Scotia Office of the Auditor General. (2016b). *Report of the Auditor General, June 2016*, chapter 2, Management of Nova Scotia's hospital system capacity. Available at http://oag-ns.ca/sites/default/files/publications/Chapter%202_0.pdf

Nusselder, W.J. (2002). *Compression of morbidity. Determining health expectancies.* Chichester: John Wiley.

O'Sullivan, B.P., Orenstein, D.M., & Milla, C.E. (2013). Pricing for orphan drugs: Will the market bear what society cannot? *Journal of the American Medical Association, 310*(13), 1343–4. https://doi.org/10.1001/jama.2013.278129

OECD. (2017a). Doctors (indicator). https://doi.org/10.1787/4355e1ec-en

OECD. (2017b). Medical graduates (indicator). https://doi.org/10.1787/ac5bd5d3-en

Office of the Chief Public Health Officer of Canada. (2008). *The Chief Public Health Officer's report on the state of public health in Canada 2008: What is public health?* Available at http://www.phac-aspc.gc.ca/cphorsphc-respcacsp/2008/fr-rc/cphorsphc-respcacsp05a-eng.php

Ontario Office of the Auditor General. (2008). *Report of the Auditor General*, chapter 3, Report on value-for-money audits. Available at http://www.auditor.on.ca/en/content/annualreports/arbyyear/ar2008.html

Pike, M., & Gibbons, C. (n.d.). Paramedic shortage: A call to action. National Human Resource Review. Available at http://0-nsleg-edeposit.gov.ns.ca .legcat.gov.ns.ca/deposit/b10657332.pdf

Power, P. (2009). E-health leads Nova Scotia's healthcare transformation. *ElectronicHealthcare*, *8*(2), e24–9.

Public Health Agency of Canada. (2011). Life with arthritis: A personal and public health challenge. Available at https://www.canada.ca/en/public -health/services/chronic-diseases/arthritis/life-arthritis-canada-a-personal -public-health-challenge/chapter-one-what-is-arthritis-and-how-common-is-it .html

Public Health Agency of Canada and CIHI. (2011). Obesity in Canada. Available at https://secure.cihi.ca/free_products/Obesity_in_canada_2011 _en.pdf

Ray, C. (2017). Loss of foreign doctor program cut at least 40 physicians from N.S. workforce. *CBC News*, 3 November 2017. Available at http://www.cbc.ca /news/canada/nova-scotia/loss-of-foreign-doctor-program-cut-more-than-40 -physicians-from-n-s-workforce-1.4384664

RBC. (2016). Canadian federal and provincial fiscal tables. Available at http:// www.rbc.com/economics/economic-reports/pdf/provincial-forecasts /prov_fiscal.pdf

Reinhardt, U. (2015). Why we should bend the cost curve and how we could do it. In G. Marchildon and L. di Matteo (Eds.), *Bending the cost curve in health care: Canada's provinces in international perspective* (pp. 3–33). Toronto: University of Toronto Press.

Requejo, F. (2010). Federalism and democracy: The case of minority nations – a federalist deficit. In M. Burgess and A. Gagnon (Eds.), *Federal democracies* (pp. 275–98). Routledge: London and New York.

Richards, J., & Busby, C. (2015). Tax burdens and the aging. In G. Marchildon and L. di Matteo (Eds.), *Bending the cost curve in health care: Canada's provinces in international perspective* (pp. 65–85). Toronto: University of Toronto Press.

Roberts, G., & Samuelson, C. (2015). *Deferred hospital maintenance in Canada*. HealthcareCAN. Available at http://www.healthcarecan.ca/wp-content/ uploads/2015/09/Deferred-Maintenance_FullDoc.pdf

Rossiter, M., Verma, J., Denis, J.L., Samis, S., Wedge, R., Power, C. (2017). Governing collaborative healthcare improvement: Lessons from an Atlantic Canadian case. *International Journal of Health Policy Management*, *6*(12), 691–4.

Ruggieri, J. (2015). Atlantic Canada: The impact of aging on the cost curve. In G. Marchildon and L. di Matteo (Eds.), *Bending the cost curve in health care: Canada's provinces in international perspective* (pp. 345–65). Toronto: University of Toronto Press.

Saillant, R. (2016). *A tale of two countries: How the great demographic imbalance is pulling Canada apart.* Halifax: Nimbus.

Savoie, D. (2015). *What is government good at?* Montreal, Kingston: McGill-Queen's University Press.

Sharif, N., Dar, A., & Amaratunga, C. (2000). *Ethnicity, income, and access to health care in the Atlantic Region: A synthesis of the literature.* Halifax: Maritime Centre of Excellence for Women's Health.

Smith, K. (2013). *Beyond evidence-based policy in public health: The interplay of ideas.* Basingstoke, UK: Palgrave-Macmillan. https://doi.org/10.1057/9781137026583

Starfield, B. (2010). Reinventing primary care: Lessons from Canada for the United States. *Health Affairs, 29*(5), 1030–6. https://doi.org/10.1377/hlthaff.2010.0002

Starfield, B., Shi, L., & Macinko, J. (2005). Contribution of primary care to health systems and health. *Health Affairs, 83*(3), 457–502.

Starr, R. (2015). Stop the silent surrender. *Nova Scotia Observer,* 25 March. Available at https://lilstar2.com/2015/03/25/stop-the-silent-surrender/

Statistics Canada. (2011a). National household survey 2011: Data tables. Available at http://www12.statcan.ca/nhs-enm/2011/dp-pd/prof/details/Page.cfm?Lang=E&Geo1=CSD&Code1=1209034&Data=Count&SearchText=Halifax&SearchType=Begins&SearchPR=01&A1=All&B1=All&GeoLevel=PR&GeoCode=10

Statistics Canada. (2011b). NHS profile, Halifax, RGM, Nova Scotia, 2011. Available at https://www12.statcan.gc.ca/nhs-enm/2011/dp-pd/prof/details/page.cfm?Lang=E&Geo1=CSD&Code1=1209034&Data=Count&SearchText=Halifax&SearchType=Begins&SearchPR=01&A1=All&B1=All&GeoLevel=PR&GeoCode=1209034&TABID=1

Statistics Canada. (2011c). Proportion (in percentage) of the population aged 65 and over, Canada, provinces and territories, 2006 and 2011. Available at https://www12.statcan.gc.ca/census-recensement/2011/as-sa/98-311-x/2011001/fig/fig7-eng.cfm

Statistics Canada. (2011d). Focus on geography series, 2011, Nova Scotia. Available at http://www12.statcan.gc.ca/census-recensement/2011/as-sa/fogs-spg/Facts-pr-eng.cfm?Lang=Eng&GC=12

Statistics Canada. (2013). Health profile, December 2013. Available at http://www12.statcan.gc.ca/health-sante/82-228/details/page.cfm?Lang=E&Tab=1&Geo1=PR&Code1=12&Geo2=PR&Code2=01&Data=Rate&SearchText=Nova%20Scotia&SearchType=Contains&SearchPR=01&B1=All&Custom=&B2=All&B3=All&GeoLevel=PR&GeoCode=12; http://novascotia.ca/dhw/publichealth/documents/Population-Health-Profile-Nova-Scotia.pdf

Statistics Canada. (2014). Estimates of population, by age group and sex for July 1, Canada, provinces and territories (CANSIM table 051–0001). Available at http://www5.statcan.gc.ca/cansim/a26?lang=eng&retrLang=eng&id=0510001&&pattern=&stByVal=1&p1=1&p2=31&tabMode=dataTable&csid=

Statistics Canada. (2016). Aboriginal peoples: Fact sheet for Nova Scotia. Available at http://www.statcan.gc.ca/pub/89-656-x/89-656-x2016004-eng.htm

Statistics Canada. (2017). Canadian health characteristics, annual estimates, by age group and sex, (Canada (excluding territories) and provinces (CANSIM table 105-0508). Available at http://www5.statcan.gc.ca/cansim/a26?lang=eng&retrLang=eng&id=1050508&pattern=&csid=

Steele, G. (2014a). *What I learned about politics.* Halifax: Nimbus.

Steele, G. (2014b). Liberals get theological on health authorities. *CBC News,* 30 January 2014. http://www.cbc.ca/news/canada/nova-scotia/graham-steele-liberals-get-theological-on-health-authorities-1.2516963

Steele, G. (2015). Health care union showdown leads to fierce political drama. *CBC* News, 23 February 2015. Available at http://www.cbc.ca/news/canada/nova-scotia/health-care-union-showdown-leads-to-fierce-political-drama-1.2968685

Steele, G. (2016). Leo Glavine shouldn't quit over pharmacare. *CBC News,* 4 February 2016. Available at http://www.cbc.ca/news/canada/nova-scotia/health-minister-resignation-pharmacare-changes-1.3433832

Stewart, M. (2001). Towards a global definition of patient centred care. *British Medical Journal, 322*(7284), 444–5. https://doi.org/10.1136/bmj.322.7284.444

Torrey, E.F., & Miller, J. (2007). *The invisible plague: The rise of mental illness from 1750 to the present.* NJ: Rutgers University Press.

Traboulsee, A., Knox, K.B., Machan, L., Zhao, Y., Yee, I., Rauscher, A., . . ., & Sadovnick, D. (2014). Prevalence of extracranial venous narrowing on catheter venography in people with multiple sclerosis, their siblings, and unrelated healthy controls: A blinded, case-control study. *Lancet, 383*(9912), 138–45. https://doi.org/10.1016/S0140-6736(13)61747-X

Tunney, C. (2015). Electronic medical record use halted in Nova Scotia hospitals. *CBC News,* 28 July 2015. Available at http://www.cbc.ca/news/canada/nova-scotia/electronic-medical-record-use-halted-in-nova-scotia-hospitals-1.3168769

Tuohy, C.H. (2003). Agency, contract, and governance: Shifting shapes of accountability in the health care arena. *Journal of Health Politics, Policy and Law, 28*(2–3), 195–215.

Twohig, P. (1991). *Health and the health care delivery system: The Micmac in Nova Scotia* (Master's thesis). St. Mary's University, Halifax, Nova Scotia.

Twohig, P. (1996). Colonial care: Medical attendance among the Mi'kmaq in Nova Scotia. *Canadian Bulletin of Medical History, 13*(2), 333–53. https://doi.org/10.3138/cbmh.13.2.333

Usher, S., Jayabarathan, A., Russell, M., & Mosher, D. (n.d.) Personal health records in primary care: One province takes steps to make sure they're available. Montreal: Health Innovation Forum.

Watson, D.E., & McGrail, K.M. (2009). More doctors or better care? *Healthcare Policy, 5*(1), 26–31.

WHO. (2015). *World report on aging and health.* Available at http://www.who.int/ageing/events/world-report-2015-launch/en/

Williams, D.R., Costa, M.V., Odunlami, A.O., & Mohammed, S.A. (2008). Moving upstream: How interventions that address the social determinants of health can improve health and reduce disparities. *Journal of Public Health Management and Practice, 14*(Suppl), S8–S17. https://doi.org/10.1097/01.PHH.0000338382.36695.42

Wiseman, N. (2007). *In search of Canadian political culture.* Vancouver: UBC Press.

Withers, P. (2015). Diana Whalen warns of worsening demographics is pre-budget speech. *CBC News*, 25 March 2015. Available at http://www.cbc.ca/news/canada/nova-scotia/diana-whalen-warns-of-worsening-demographics-in-pre-budget-speech-1.3008968

Wong, J. (2014). Debate flies over move to regulate private healthcare industry in N.S. *Global News*, 17 June 2014. Available at http://globalnews.ca/news/1399819/debate-flies-over-move-to-regulate-private-healthcare-industry-in-n-s/

Workers' Compensation Board of Nova Scotia. (2015). Workplace injury insurance (website). http://wcb.ns.ca/Workplace-Injury-Insurance/Benefits-of-Coverage.aspx

Yoshikawa, H., Aber, J.L., & Beardslee, W.R. (2012). The effects of poverty on the mental, emotional, and behavioral health of children and youth: Implications for prevention. *American Psychologist, 67*(4), 272–84. https://doi.org/10.1037/a0028015

Index

rationale, 151, 159; shared service area (SSA) model, 121
Diversity and Inclusion Steering Committee, 175
doctors. *See* physicians
Doctors Nova Scotia. *See* Nova Scotia Medical Society
Dorsey, James, 155–7
Drug Evaluation Alliance of Nova Scotia (DEANS), 133
Drug Information System (DIS), 81, 87–8, 134
Duckett, S., 167

economy, 7–10; debt levels, 8; employment, 9–10; federal transfers, 7, 8, 62–3, *65*, 68–9; future possibilities, 10; GDP, 8, *9*; history, 7–8; investment, 9; labour force decline, 8–9; tax rates and revenue, 61, *65*, 172–*3*; trade, 10
education. *See* Dalhousie University and Medical School
efficiency, 183–5, 191
811 service. *See* telehealth service
electrolysis, 48
electronic health information systems: introduction, 80–1; ANDS system, 123; assessment of, 177; Client and Provider Registries, 83; Computerized Physician Order Entry system, 88; Drug Information System (DIS), 81, 87–8, 134; electronic health records (EHRs), 81–3, 88; electronic medical records (EMRs), 81, 83–4, *85–6*; Emergency Department Information System, 88; Food and Nutrition Services (FaNS), 86–7; need to reform, 196; Nova Scotia hospital Information

System (NShIS), 81–2, 87, 88; One Person, One Record system, 88, 161, 164, 185; organizational structure, *82*; Panorama program, 88–9, 123, 124; Patient Access Registry Nova Scotia (PAR-NS), 81, 87, 126, 171; patient flow system, 87; personal health records (PHRs), 81, 84, 86, 187; Picture Archiving Communications System (PACS), 81, 83, 180; Primary Health Care Information Management (PHIM), 81, 83; public health challenges, 123–4; responsibility for, 43, 160–1; Secure Health Access Record (SHARE), 82–3, 88, 177; Telehealth Network, 86
electronic health records (EHRs), 81–3, 88
electronic medical records (EMRs), 81, 83–4, *85–6*
Emergency Department Information System, 88
emergency health services, 127–30; administration, 128–9; assessment of, 177; components, 128; costs and financing, 64, 129; history, 127–8; reform efforts, 129–30. *See also* ambulance services; paramedics
Emergency Health Services (EHS), 41, 127
Emergency Medical Care Inc. (EMC), 41, 128–9
employment, 3, 9–10. *See also* health human resources
Employment Insurance, 4–5
environmental public health professionals, *98, 99*
epidemics, 2, 16, 17
epidemiologists, 123

www.ingramcontent.com/pod-product-compliance
Lightning Source LLC
Chambersburg PA
CBHW030240030426
42336CB00009B/181